Perfect Body
STYLING

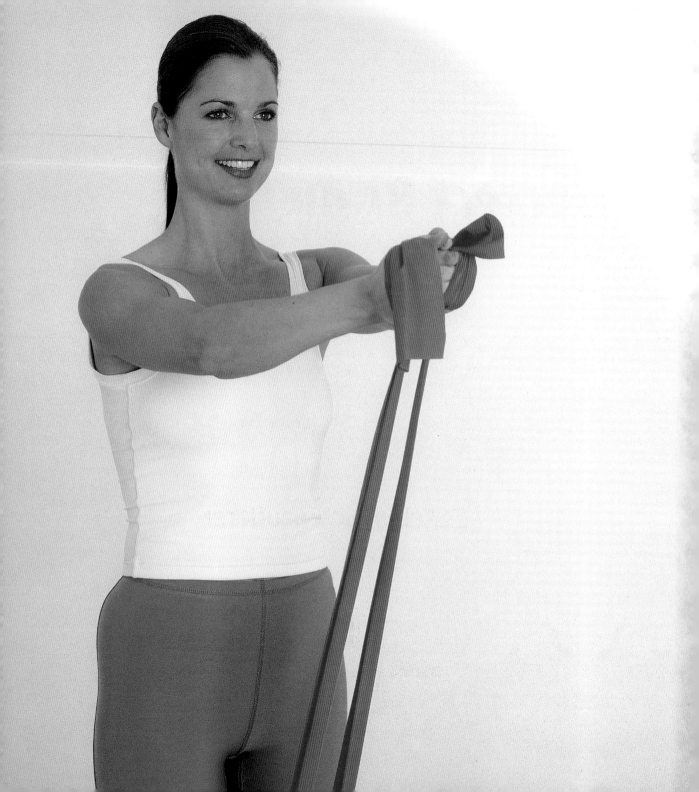

Perfect Body
STYLING

Heiko Czichoschewski

Wolfgang Mießner

Achim Schmauderer

Sterling Publishing Co., Inc.
New York

Photo credits

All photographs by Susanne Kracke,
   except:

p. 6, 20, 120, 143, 145, 153, 161,
   163, 168, 170, 174, 176, 178 by
   Ulli Seer

p.147 by Chili Photography (Andreas
   Meier)

p. 148 left, by Adidas

p.148 right, 155, 156, 158, 160, 162,
   167, 181, 182 by Polar

p.149, 177 by Oryk Haist

p.150 by Odlo

p.154, 159 by Dominik Parzinger

p.171, 172, 173 by Konopka Archive

p.180 by Illuscope

Illustrations on pages 12, 13, 15, 16
   by Jörg Mair

*Translated from the German by
Maria-Theresia Holub*

Library of Congress Cataloging-in-Publication Data Available

1 0 9 8 7 6 5 4 3 2 1

Published in 2006 by Sterling Publishing Co., Inc.
387 Park Avenue South, New York, NY 10016
Originally published in Germany under the title *Perfect Body Styling*
by BLV Verlagsgesellschaft mbH, Postfach 4013 20, 80703 München
The authors are Heiko Czichoschewski, Wolfgang Mießner, and Achim Schmauderer
Copyright © 2004 by BLV Verlagsgesellschaft mbH
English Translation Copyright © 2006 by Sterling Publishing Co., Inc.
Distributed in Canada by Sterling Publishing
c/o Canadian Manda Group, 165 Dufferin Street
Toronto, Ontario, Canada M6K 3H6
Distributed in the United Kingdom by GMC Distribution Services,
Castle Place, 166 High Street, Lewes, East Sussex, England BN7 1XU
Distributed in Australia by Capricorn Link (Australia) Pty Ltd.
P.O. Box 704, Windsor, NSW 2756, Australia

Manufactured in China
All Rights Reserved

Sterling ISBN-13: 978-1-4027-3097-9
Sterling ISBN-10: 1-4027-3097-7

For information about custom editions, special sales, premium and
corporate purchases, please contact Sterling Special Sales
Department at 800-805-5489 or specialsales@sterlingpub.com.

Contents

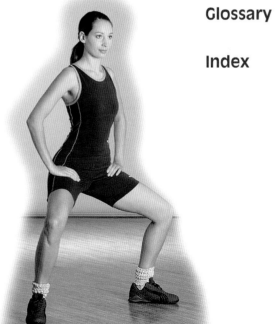

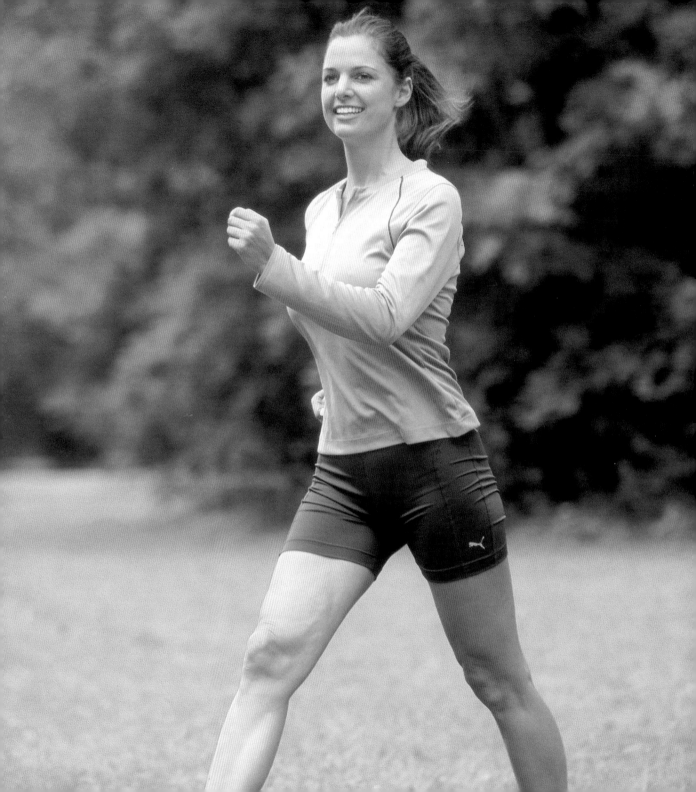

Introduction
Body Styling:
Shaping the Body

Body styling is a gentle way of shaping the body. It consists of specific muscle training with light to medium weights, as well as cardiovascular training (also known as "endurance sports"). But Body Styling is even more; it includes keeping to a healthy diet and body care. It is this combination that helps you have a body you feel comfortable with. Toned muscles are not just a matter of aesthetics; increased muscle strength is also good for your health. Today we move far too little or too inadequately in our everyday lives. The World Health Organization recommends either 30 minutes of exercise daily or participating in a sport 3–4 times a week. Through a lack of movement, muscles become weak and inflexible. The consequences are pain and structural imbalance of the spine. This can be prevented through a balanced Body Styling program. The most important part of Body Styling is a fitness workout that consists of one or two types of endurance sports plus muscle training. Which endurance sports you choose depends on your individual preference. Sports scientists call the muscle training in Body Styling "strength endurance workout." This workout creates strengthened tissue and a heightened metabolism which enables you to burn calories more quickly—a good prerequisite for dealing with possible weight problems.

In this book you will first find some basics of anatomy. You will then receive tips for a general workout. These are followed by exercises to strengthen your muscles. The exercises are presented according to individual body zones, starting with the shoulders and arms, moving on to the back, the problem zones of the abdomen and buttocks, and down to the legs. The subsequent section focuses on burning fat and on endurance workouts, followed by sections on nutrition, relaxation, and wellness.

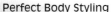

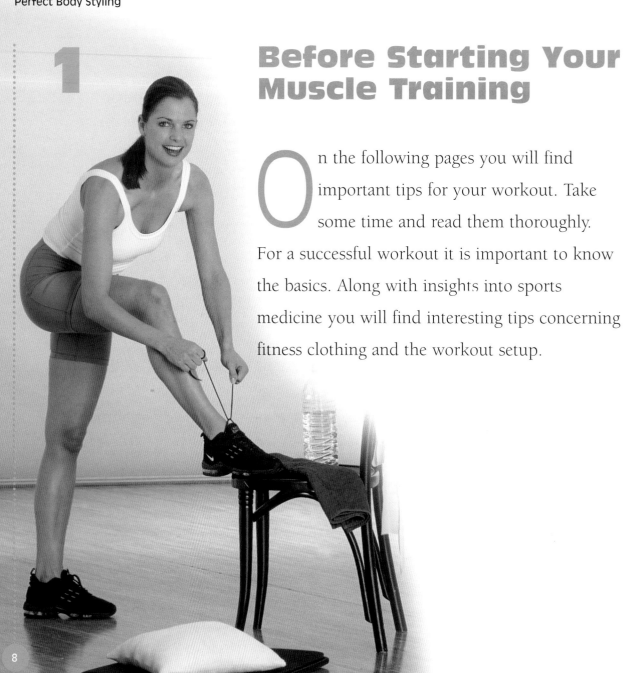

1

Before Starting Your Muscle Training

On the following pages you will find important tips for your workout. Take some time and read them thoroughly. For a successful workout it is important to know the basics. Along with insights into sports medicine you will find interesting tips concerning fitness clothing and the workout setup.

General Workout Advice

Before starting your workout, please pay attention to the following points:

- Wear comfortable clothes, such as sweatpants and a T-shirt. Avoid tight-fitting garments.
- Remove all jewelry.

> As a beginner, you should not put too much strain on your muscles. Do not exercise daily; give yourself a day of rest. Beginners should work out a maximum of 2—3 days per week. In between you may do regenerative stretching or take a sauna in order to relax as well as to increase your overall well-being.

Tips

- Running, fast walking in place, or cycling are especially recommended for warming up. The warm-up should last at least 5 minutes.
- Start exercising in front of a mirror so that you gain more firm control over your posture.

- Wear sneakers.
- Set out a mat, a pillow for your head, and a towel.
- Prepare a drink for your break. Tip: If you mix juice and water 1:1 you will have a drink that is both tasty and healthy. Make sure it is not too cold.
- Try to avoid distractions. For instance, switch on your answering machine and switch off your cell phone.
- Listen to your favorite music during your workout.

Specific Workout Advice

- Always warm up. This protects you from injury and stimulates your circulation.
- Pay attention to your starting position and revise it if necessary.
- Concentrate on your breathing and the correct performance of the exercises. Lack of concentration increases the risk of injury.

- Repeat exercises 10–15 times. This equals one set. Do 2–4 sets of each exercise and practice 2–3 times a week. One workout session with a warm-up and a cool-down should last at least 30 minutes.
- Add variety to your workout. Change exercises every 4–6 weeks. Always choose exercises for various muscle groups.
- The best workout time is between 4 p.m. and 8 p.m. If you want to exercise early in the morning you should warm up very thoroughly.
- Avoid working out after 9 p.m., as exercise can cause troubled sleep.

You should not work out if you have:
- an infection, the flu, or indigestion
- a fever
- acute pain
- a poor overall physical condition
- taken medication or drunk alcohol

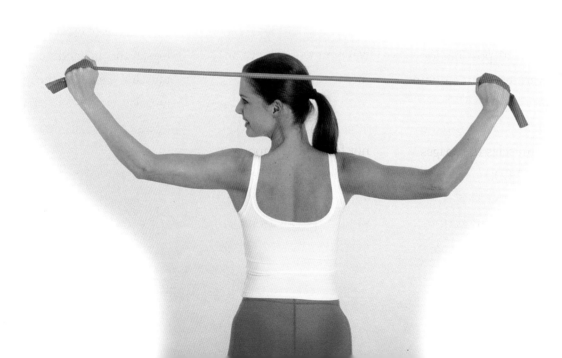

Tip

If you had your last physical more than six months ago you should see your doctor for another checkup. This way potential problems can be noticed in time.

Workout Systems

There are different methods to choose for your workout:

- General fitness: This form of workout focuses on flexibility and strength. You exercise 2–3 times a week, doing as many exercises as possible for the various muscle groups. Following strength training you will stretch your muscles (see pages 118 to 142).
- Building up muscles: If you specifically want to build up muscle mass, you must isolate the different muscle groups, concentrating on certain muscle groups in one workout session. On subsequent days you will choose different muscle groups to work on. This way you will achieve an intensive buildup of muscle. Make sure to have a balanced workout. Do not forget any important muscles! For the very ambitious, work on the same muscle with no pause between two sets. Choose two different exercises for this. You will immediately feel a highly increased circulation in your tissue.
- Increasing flexibility: If your workout goal is greater flexibility then the following method is right for you. Stretch those muscle groups whose flexibility needs to be improved. Choose exercises accordingly.
- After doing the strengthening exercise, loosen the affected muscles. This way the muscles are relaxed after being contracted.

Tip

Take as much time building muscle as stretching.

An Excursion into Anatomy

When planning your workout it is important to know the individual muscle groups. Let's start with the legs. On the lower thigh we have two significant muscle groups, the anterior and posterior calf muscles. The posterior calf muscles (*M. gastrocnemius*) enable us to stand erect. This muscle group is also particularly important for the so-called vein pump. The anterior

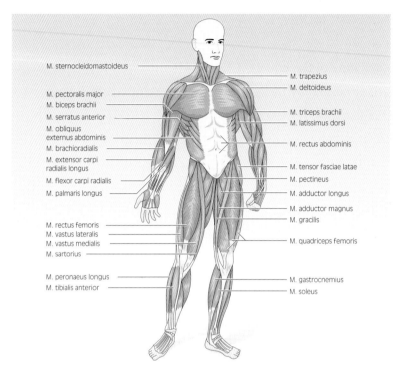

M. sternocleidomastoideus
M. pectoralis major
M. biceps brachii
M. serratus anterior
M. obliquus externus abdominis
M. brachioradialis
M. extensor carpi radialis longus
M. flexor carpi radialis
M. palmaris longus
M. rectus femoris
M. vastus lateralis
M. vastus medialis
M. sartorius
M. peronaeus longus
M. tibialis anterior

M. trapezius
M. deltoideus
M. triceps brachii
M. latissimus dorsi
M. rectus abdominis
M. tensor fasciae latae
M. pectineus
M. adductor longus
M. adductor magnus
M. gracilis
M. quadriceps femoris
M. gastrocnemius
M. soleus

Surface skeletal muscles, front view.

Tip

The vein pump assists your heart. Through contraction of the calf muscles blood is pumped actively into the heart.

lower thigh muscles (*M. tibialis anterior*) enable us to walk heel-to-toe. If you lack strength in your legs, you will appear to waddle. On the upper thigh's anterior you have a thigh muscle consisting of four parts (*M. quadriceps femoris*) that flexes the hip and extends the knee. The so-called adductors are located on the inner thighs.

When you pull your leg

toward your body, the bending of the knee and stretching of the hip are accomplished by the hamstrings (*M. biceps femoris, M. semitendinosus*, and *M. semimembranosus*) at the back of your upper thighs.

The gluteal (buttocks) muscles (*M. glutaeus*), which are involved in all movements of the hip joints, stretch from the exterior of the upper thighs down to the lower thighs. The abdominal muscles consist of, among others, the straight abdominal muscle (*M. rectus abdominis*), which forms the famous "six-pack." The oblique abdominal muscles (*M. obliquus externus abdominis*) and the *transversus abdominis* muscle

complete the bracing of the anterior abdominal wall. Abdominal muscles are an important factor in your physical stability. Above the abdomen lie the pectoral (chest) muscles. They consist of major and minor pectorals

(*M. pectorales* major and minor). This muscle group is hardly one to be troubled over nowadays. It is activated only when you wash your hands or shake out a blanket.

Daily use of these muscles was lost when people started

Skeletal muscles, back view.

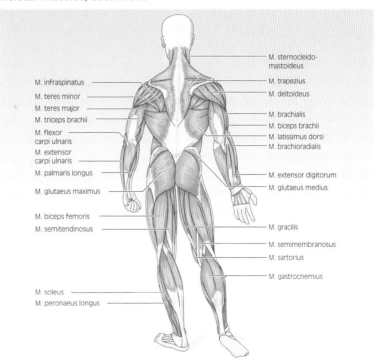

M. infraspinatus
M. teres minor
M. teres major
M. triceps brachii
M. flexor carpi ulnaris
M. extensor carpi ulnaris
M. palmaris longus
M. glutaeus maximus
M. biceps femoris
M. semitendinosus
M. soleus
M. peronaeus longus

M. sternocleido-mastoideus
M. trapezius
M. deltoideus
M. brachialis
M. biceps brachii
M. latissimus dorsi
M. brachioradialis
M. extensor digitorum
M. glutaeus medius
M. gracilis
M. semimembranosus
M. sartorius
M. gastrocnemius

to walk upright. Among animals that move on all fours, the pectorals play an important role. (Caution: In case of stiffness in the neck, the pectorals need to be stretched well!)

The back muscles are subdivided into deep and surface muscles. The deep back muscles consist of a complex group of muscles that are responsible for correct posture. The surface muscles (*M. latissimus dorsi*) on the other hand perform large movements. For instance, the strength of the shoulder derives in large part from the back muscles. The head is stabilized by the neck and throat muscles. A number of smaller and larger muscles accomplish this

task. Many problems in the area of the shoulders and neck are caused by these muscles. Weakness or tension both lead to discomfort, with symptoms ranging from simple stiffness to migraine headaches. For this reason it is vitally important to train these muscle groups.

The deltoids or shoulder

Tip

In cases of "tennis arm," one of the lower arm extensors is usually overly strained. Causes can be either frequent tennis playing or hard physical labor. You can relieve the pain through light arm exercises and through cooling the affected area.

muscles (*M. deltoideus*) are crucial to the overall posture of the body. Just as the glutes perform all movement at the hip, the deltoids are involved in all movements of the shoulder. The arm muscles are less important for posture. They should be strong enough to carry daily loads without problems. They are subdivided into upper arm and lower arm muscles. On the upper arm the flexors (*M. biceps brachii*) are in the front, and the extensors (*M. triceps brachii*) in the back. Hand and finger strength derive from the lower arm, where a similar subdivision can be discerned: the flexors lie on the lower side, and the extensors on the upper side.

Body Types

The human body is for the most part determined by genes. This includes height, bone structure, and joint structure. Working out cannot influence any of these features, but it can influence factors such as posture and the amount of fatty tissue in your body. Anatomists like to make a subdivision of physical conformation into three different types. Try to find out which type you belong to. No one actually resembles one type 100 percent. Normally, every person is a mixture of these three types.

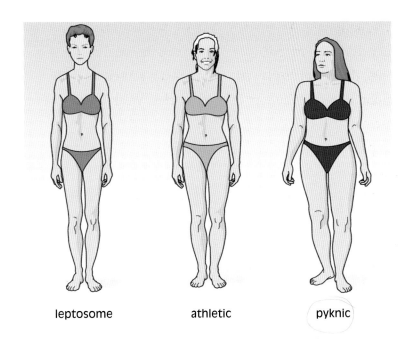

leptosome　　　　athletic　　　　pyknic

The Leptosome or Ectomorphic Type

Leptosomes are long-limbed. They appear slight and have thin shoulders. Bones stand out distinctly and the amount of fatty tissue in the body is low. The rather active metabolism quickly processes food, so that these people can eat without gaining a lot of weight. Oftentimes leptosomes tend to slouch a bit, which makes muscle training all the more important for them to balance faulty posture. Although leptosomes appear less sporty, they can build up muscles through systematic training.

The Athletic or Mesomorphic Type

Strong bone structure, strong joints, and a muscular build characterize persons of this type. Chest and shoulders are especially wide; the pelvis, by contrast, is rather small. Especially at the lower limbs of arms and legs the muscles are built strongly. Mostly men belong to this type. Athletic people easily build up muscle mass but do not necessarily have the ideal prerequisites for endurance sports such as long-distance running. Weight problems are usually unknown to them.

The Pyknic or Endomorphic Type

The pyknic type is prone to a rounder figure; the layer of fatty tissue is more developed than in the other two types and bones do not stand out. Fat pads may appear in the midsection of the body and on the legs. Metabolism is rather slow, which leads easily to weight gain. Women belong to this type much more often than men. Endurance workout and systematic strength exercises will stimulate metabolism and increase fat burning—a healthy diet is also very important.

Apple or Pear?

Fat is stored by both sexes because the body creates a

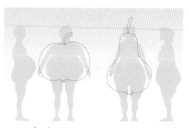

apple type   pear type

fat supply for "hard times." Lack of nutrition is hardly part of our modern-day societies anymore, except when dieting. Women build up a subcutaneous layer of fat on the buttocks and upper thighs, leading to "saddle bags," while men store fat in the stomach, which leads to a "beer belly." Since this different storage of fat causes different physical types, men are often called apple types whereas women are called pear types.

The Balanced Workout Program

In order to perform a health-oriented and effective workout, keep in mind the following points: During a workout session always train both agonist (the main mobility muscle) and antagonist (the opposite muscle). For toning your arms this means the agonist is the biceps and the antagonist is the triceps. The same principle applies to the chest (agonist) and the upper and midsection of the back (antagonist). Studies in sports medicine have shown that one should train the chest and back in a ratio of 2:3. For the upper part of the shoulder (agonist) the antagonist is the rear part of your shoulder muscle. One-sided training can lead to muscle imbalance! Evasive, compensatory movements resulting from this procedure negatively affect other muscles and joints.

You will find exercises for your back on page 52, and exercises for your abdomen on page 70. Choose one exercise for each muscle group. In order not to stress your circulation too much, you should first perform all strength exercises standing up and then lying down. This will also help with stretching, because after the last strength-training exercise on the floor you can relax with stretching exercises.

Frequency of Training

For beginners, a workout frequency of 2–3 times a week is recommended. In between you should take periods of rest, because fitness decreases during workout. A real increase in fitness is only possible after a period of rest. An overzealous attitude and the idea that "a lot will change a lot" will not yield good results and can actually be harmful to both your physical and mental fitness in the long run. By all means grant yourself rest periods or include an active day of relaxation, such as stretching or taking a walk.

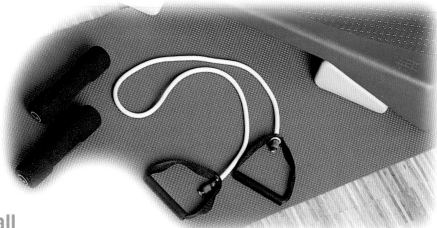

Using Small Fitness Gear

Thera-Band resistive exercise bands and exercise tubing are available in different colors. Each color signifies a particular tractive force. From "extra light" to "extra heavy" the right band is available for everyone. If you have never worked with a Thera-Band before, start with an extra light or light.

Small hand weights can be purchased in different sizes and weights. For beginners we recommend weights from 2–6 pounds (1–3 kilograms) per piece.

Exercise handles (handles connected to a resistive tube) are a great conditioning tool and can be used in many exercises.

Some exercises are performed on a step, but if you do not have this piece of equipment you can exercise on the floor or use a sturdy footstool instead.

Tip

As an alternative to hand weights, you can also use plastic bottles filled with either water or sand.

Safety Advice

■ Take some time to go through your workout. Plan at least 30 minutes for your exercises and take your own fitness level into account.

■ If you choose to do exercises with Thera-Bands and exercise handles, check before starting the workout that the tubing is not torn. Make sure the tubes have not been knotted or exposed to direct sunlight or heating.

■ Even if you are in a hurry, never leave out the warm-up (stretching before the workout) or the cool-down (stretching at the end of the workout).

■ For all exercises on the floor, use an exercise mat and a towel or blanket to keep the impact on bones and joints as low as possible.

■ To prevent injury avoid abrupt movements. Perform the exercises in a smooth, strong, controlled, and, above all, slow manner.

■ Never hold your breath during exercise and avoid pressure breathing. Breathe slowly and evenly; exhale while tightening your muscles and inhale while relaxing them.

■ For exercises with Thera-Bands, make sure that they are always tight and never sag. This guarantees an effective training, because a slight basic tension within the muscles can always be discerned.

■ The knee and elbow joints should remain slightly bent in the standing, lying, or holding position.

■ Between individual exercises, add 20–30 seconds of rest so that you gently loosen the affected muscles.

10 Good Reasons to Exercise

- Increases resistance against external forces

- Improves posture and body control

- Prevents muscle imbalance or equalizes an existing imbalance

- Protects joints and other sensitive body parts against injury

- Increases burning of calories, which decreases fat mass and helps define muscles

- Slows down the aging process

- Increases muscle tone

- Improves circulation

- Increased strength helps you deal better with the stress of daily life

- Increased bone density helps prevent osteoporosis

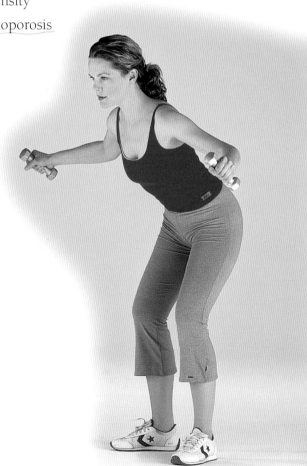

Safe and Effective Exercises for Everyone

- All exercises in this book are geared toward functionality and health. Please consider your own fitness level when selecting exercises.

- For beginners it is recommended that you do all the basic exercises with only one set per exercise. Once you are able to perform the movements correctly, you are ready for the next level: the variation exercises. For advanced exercisers we recommend you do 2–3 sets of the selected exercises with 15–20 repetitions.

- For each workout session design your own personal program so that you stay motivated and do not get bored. Soon you will find your favorite exercises to use for your workout.

- The warm-up at the beginning of your workout and the cool-down at the end complete your workout program.

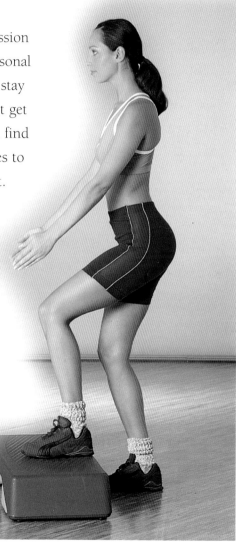

Practical Advice

Your workout should be not only successful, but also fun. If the basic prerequisites are met, you will always look forward to your training and exercise enthusiastically.

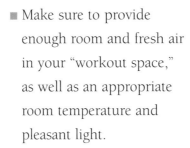

■ Make sure to provide enough room and fresh air in your "workout space," as well as an appropriate room temperature and pleasant light.

■ The choice of clothing is up to you. It is important that you feel comfortable and have enough room to move. Solid footwear is a must in order to prevent injuries during warm-up and during standing exercises or exercises involving Thera-Bands.

■ Switch off your phones so that you can concentrate on your workout without any distractions.

■ Put all devices such as Thera-Bands, chairs, or exercise mats within reach.

■ Prepare a thirst-quenching drink for yourself.

■ Have a towel within reach for when you have worked up a sweat.

■ With music everything works more easily; put on your favorite CD and turn up the volume of your stereo or walkman to an agreeable level.

The following workout session is just for you. Use the time as effectively as possible.

2   Now Let's Get Started!

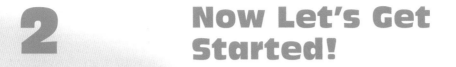

On the following pages you will find the appropriate exercises for your individual workout. Choose a program that you can perform several times a week. You only need some small fitness gear and the motivation to change your body to your own advantage. Just start! You will soon feel and see the successful results.

23

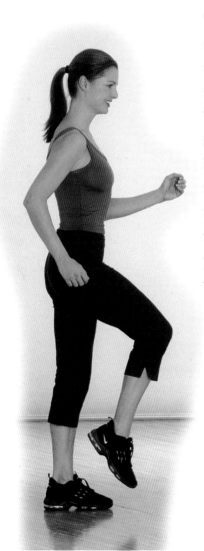

Warm-Up

The warm-up is a very important workout phase that should never be forgotten or neglected. Through the warm-up you activate your body. Your heart rate and breathing rate increase and your body temperature rises. This increase in body heat helps prevent injuries during your workout.

Walking

- Walk in place. Start at a slow tempo. Move your arms rhythmically. Breathe slowly and evenly.
- After a few minutes increase your tempo. Swing your arms faster and lift your feet off the floor.

For walking, wear sneakers to protect your joints. The risk of injury is very high if you are barefoot, especially on soft surfaces.

Jumping rope

- Make some room for yourself and take your rope in both hands.
- Now swing the rope over your head and when it comes back down jump over it with both feet. You can choose between two options: jump with both feet simultaneously, or skip. The first option is a bit more strenuous and burns additional calories.

Cycling

- If you have a treadmill or other equipment available, you can use it for warm-up.
- Start with low resistance, which you may slowly increase after a few

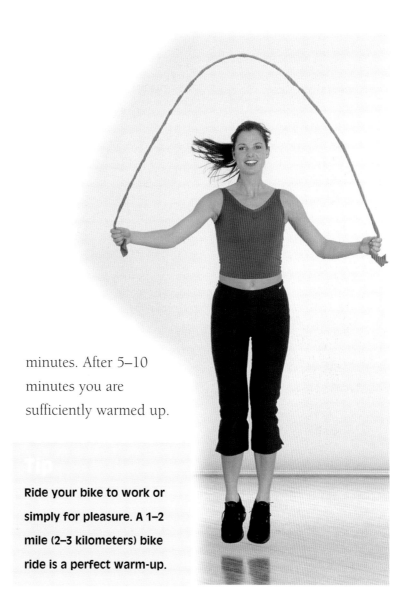

minutes. After 5–10 minutes you are sufficiently warmed up.

Ride your bike to work or simply for pleasure. A 1–2 mile (2–3 kilometers) bike ride is a perfect warm-up.

Info

The warm-up is divided into three phases:

1. The general warm-up serves to increase the body core temperature, which should rise to about 101.3 to 102.2 degrees Fahrenheit (38.5 to 39 degrees Celsius) to guarantee maximum speed of metabolic processes. Light to medium stress through jogging is sufficient.

2. The individual warm-up depends on personal preference but also on existing limitations of the person working out (e.g., handicapped or injured).

3. The specific warm-up depends on the specific kind of impact on the joints and helps to mobilize the affected joints.

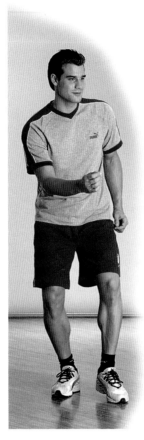

"Out-out, In-in"

- Starting from a "walking" position, alternately open and close your legs.

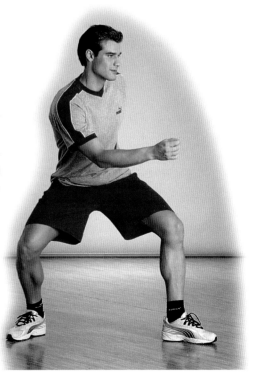

Step Touch

- Stand upright with your legs closed. With your right leg, take a step to the side. Quickly follow with your left foot and tap the floor with your toe.

- Alternately perform this step to the left and to the right side.

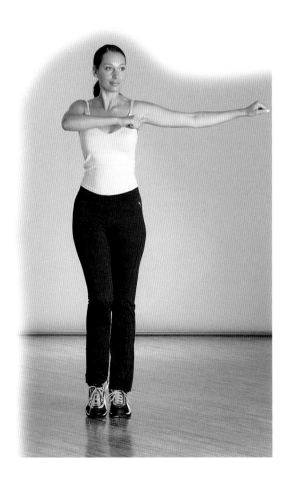
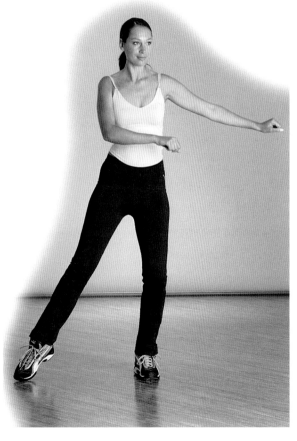

Heel Dig

- Stand upright and alternately move your left and right heel to the front and quickly touch the floor.
- During this exercise extend your arms almost straight in front of you and lift them up to your shoulders with strength and control. Then lower them again.
- Keep your knees bent at all times.

Make sure that your torso remains stabilized during the whole exercise. Do not step backward.

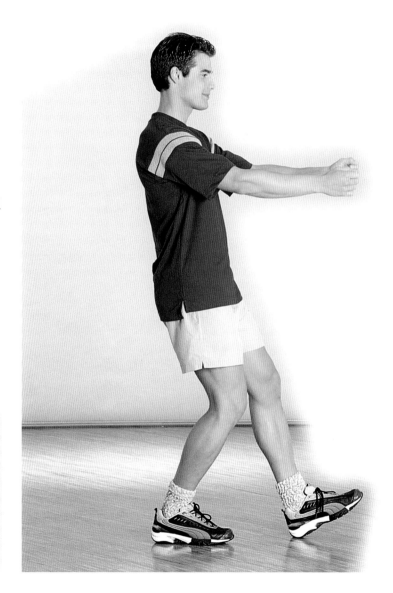

Side to Side

- Stand with your legs apart and balance your weight on your right leg. With your left foot tap the floor with your toe.
- Move back to the middle, lower your leg, and perform the movement with the weight on your left leg.
- Keep your knees bent at all times.

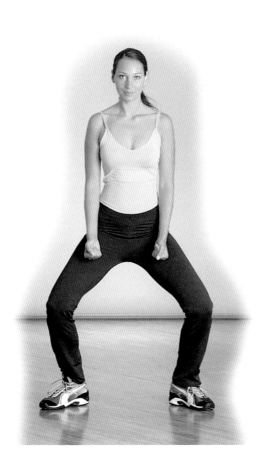

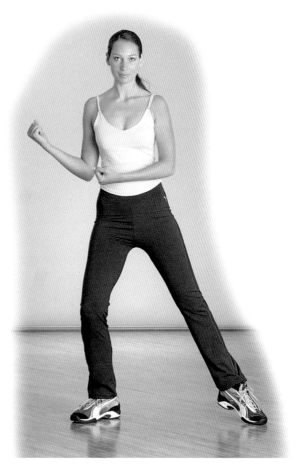

Toe Tap

- Stand upright with legs closed and slightly bent. Cross your arms in front of your body.

- Alternately tap your left and right foot to the side.
- With some strength, lift your arms sideways up to your shoulders.

- During the whole exercise keep your shoulders relaxed and pulled down. Gently clench your fists.

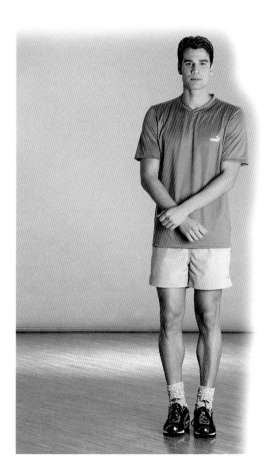
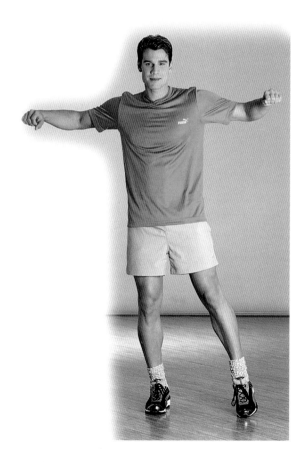

Joint isolation exercises

Shoulder Rotation

- Stand in an upright position with your legs shoulder-width apart. Now slowly "paint" a circle with your shoulders. Repeat this forward movement several times and then change direction.

- You can also perform this exercise individually, that is, first rotate your right shoulder, then your left.

Chest Opener

- Stand upright and lift your arms until the elbows reach up to the shoulders. The forearms and upper arms now form an angle of about 90 degrees. Your palms should be facing forward.

- Move your arms back and inhale and exhale deeply. Pull your shoulder blades down.

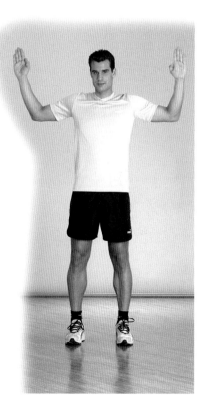

Info

Apart from exercises that involve your whole body, which mainly serve to increase the body core temperature, there are also joint isolation exercises. You will find these exercises on the following page. Joint isolation exercises are geared toward mobilizing the body and preparing the joints for wider movements. Perform these exercises slowly and in place.

If you want to do exercises with medium to heavy weights, you should add a specific warm-up in which you perform a set of exercises with light weights.

Back Isolation

Stand upright with your legs shoulder-width apart. Bend your torso forward and stabilize it by putting your hands on your upper thighs. Your head forms an extension of your spine. Now arch your back and then slowly lower your back again until it is in an upright position.

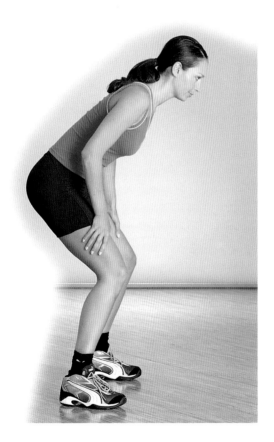

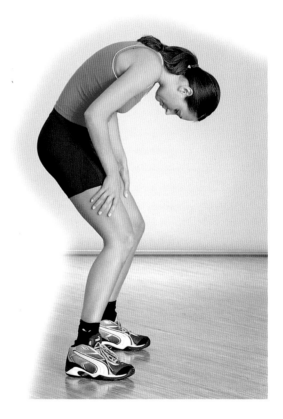

3

Styling for Your Body!

Are you unhappy with certain areas of your body? With these workout exercises you can systematically tone individual body zones. You will strengthen your muscles and lift tissue if you perform the exercises on a regular basis.

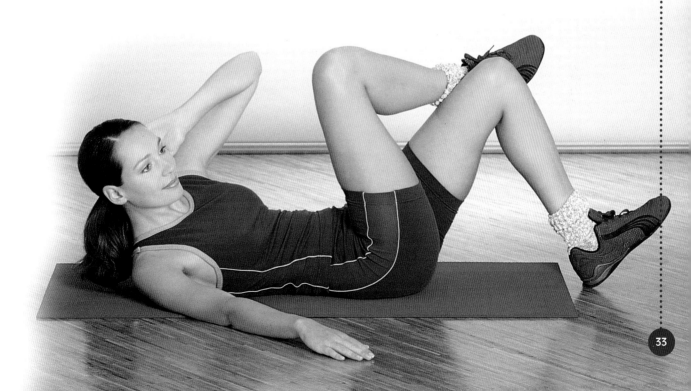

Strength Training for Your Arms

Beautiful arms are also part of a harmonious build and complete the appearance of the upper body. The "flexor" of the arm, also called the biceps, makes up essentially the front side of the upper arm. In fitness studios it is usually men who train this muscle. The antagonist of the biceps is the triceps, which form the outer side of the upper arm. The fears of some women that they will appear too masculine and bulky from training their arms are completely unfounded. Ongoing practice with medium resistance tones the muscles and tissue—your arms will look firm and defined, but not bulky.

Biceps Curls

■ For this exercise you can choose the degree of difficulty through your starting position: walking position = light, standing position with legs closed = medium, standing position with legs open = difficult. Choose your preferred position according to your fitness level.

■ Place your foot in the

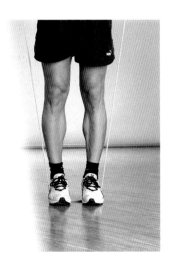
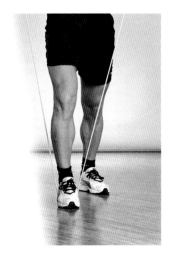
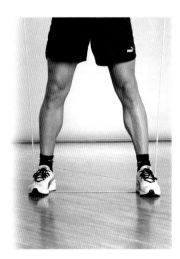

middle of the rubber tube or exercise handle.

- Grab the handles, with palms facing up. Hold your elbows close in to your body during the whole exercise. Your forearms should form a straight line with your hands.

- Pull your shoulders down while flexing and extending your arms at the elbows.

Variation

- As an alternative to tubing or exercise handles, you can use hand weights for this exercise.

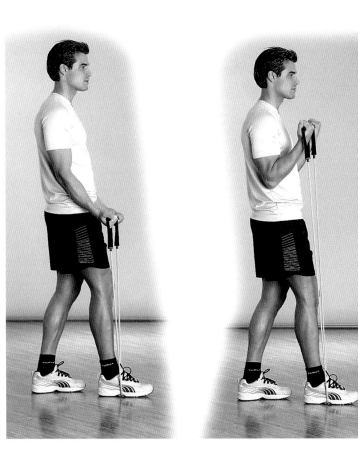

Info

Hold your torso upright at all times. Leaning your upper body back will place too much pressure on your lower back.

Sitting Biceps Curls with One Arm

- Sit down on a step bench or a footstool and open your legs wide. With your back straight, lean your torso slightly forward. Place the elbow of your right arm on your right inner thigh. Support the other hand with your left upper thigh. Make sure to keep your shoulders pulled down and relaxed.
- Slowly flex and extend your arm. Always keep contact between your elbow and your upper thigh and tighten your biceps.
- Afterward, perform this exercise with the other arm.

Info

You should hold the hand weights with your wrist in neutral position.

Standing Triceps

- Stand upright, with your back straight and your legs shoulder-width apart.
- Loosely tie the tube around your hand so that the band shortens and forms a loop.

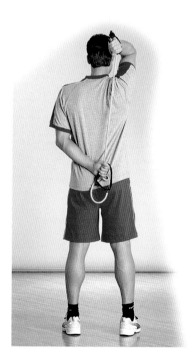

- With one hand, place the tube above your buttocks. Your other arm should be extended over your head with your elbow pointing to the ceiling.

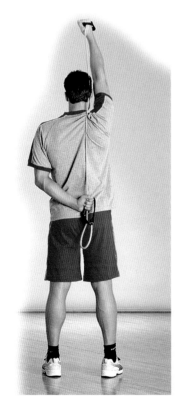

Info

It is very important to keep the tubing tight. Even when you are in starting position, the tube should not sag.

- Now extend and flex the upper arm. Keep your wrists straight throughout the entire exercise and your shoulders pulled down.
- Afterward, repeat the exercise with the other arm the same number of times.

Variation

- You can also perform this exercise lying on your stomach.
- Open your legs shoulder width-apart and rest your feet on your toes. Slightly tighten your buttocks.
- For this exercise keep your torso as close as possible to the floor to avoid swaying.

Tip

To support your pelvis place a rolled-up towel under your hips.

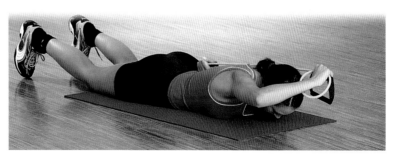

Upward Walking Triceps

- Stand in walking position, legs parallel. The knees of both legs remain slightly bent. Place the tube under your back foot. Keep your back and torso straight and your shoulders pulled down. You should now form a solid line from head to toe. Make sure you do not lean back during the exercise.

- If you stand on the tube with your left foot, work with your right arm, and vice versa. The wrist of the active arm remains stabilized as an extension of your forearm. With the other hand, support the arm and hold the elbow of the moving arm close to your head and pointing to the ceiling.

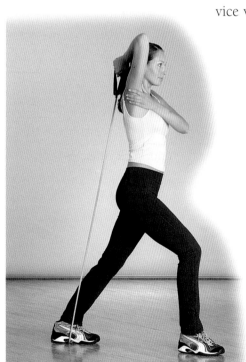
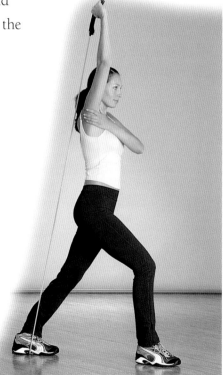

- Now lift up your lower arm. Make sure not to overstretch your elbow.
- During this exercise do not forget to reverse your arms and legs.

Variation A

- You can also perform this exercise with hand weights.

Variation B

- You can also perform this exercise with the tube while sitting.
- For this purpose place the tube under the leg of a chair. Make sure to keep your back straight and

stabilized during the exercise. Keep your legs slightly open for better stabilization of your body. You may also use hand weights.

- This exercise and its variants train the shoulder and neck muscles.

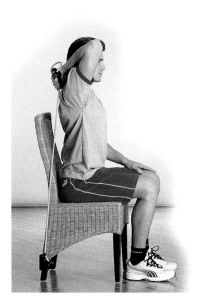

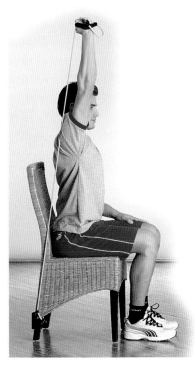

Triceps Kickback

- With one leg, kneel on the step bench. Place the other leg on the floor so that it forms a vertical line from knee to foot.

- Support your body in the front with one hand on the step and keep your back straight. The head forms an extension from the torso.

- The other arm holds the hand weight; keep it bent and close to your body.

- Using your elbow, extend and flex your arm.

- Afterward, repeat the exercise with your other arm.

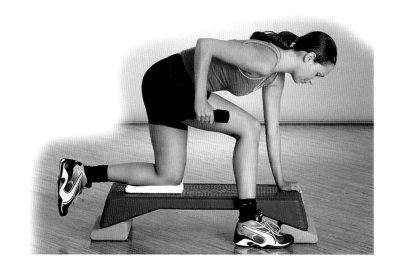

Tip

To reduce pressure on the knees you should put a towel or exercise mat underneath.

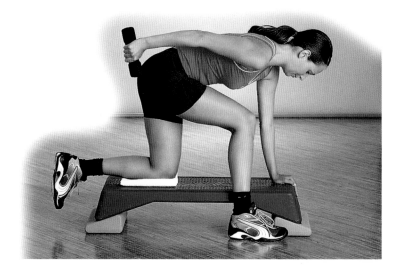

French Press

- Lie down with your head and back on the step. Place one bent leg on the floor and place the other knee on top of it.
- Hold one hand weight in each hand. Your elbows and palms should face the ceiling and form a straight line with your shoulders.
- Lift up your forearms without leaning your elbows to the front or the side.
- Flex your arms and move back to the starting position.

Tip

If you are prone to swaying, simply pull up your knees to your body.

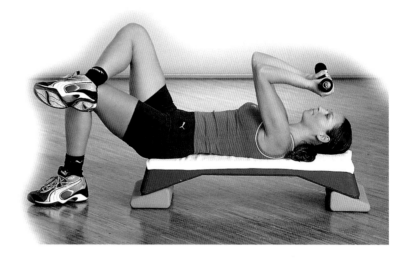

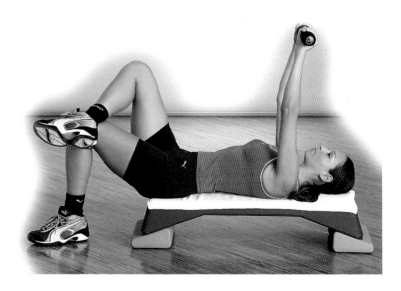

Tip

Depending on your fitness level, you may change the basic resistance of the Thera-Band by holding it either tightly or loosely.

Thera-Band Arm Extension

- Hold the Thera-Band exercise band behind your head. Bend your upper arm and forearm into a 90-degree angle.
- Alternately extend one arm against the resistance of the band.

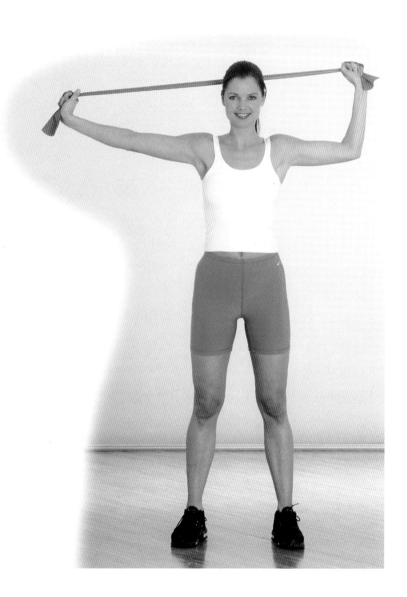

Kickback with Exercise Handles

Starting position:

- Standing in a walking position, bend your front leg and secure the tube with your foot. Lean your torso forward with your back and rear leg forming a straight line.
- The active arm holds the tube on one end and is raised so that the elbow points away from your torso. Your palms are facing the body.
- The inactive arm holds the other end of the tube and rests on the upper thigh.

Execution of the exercise:

- Move the active arm backward without overstretching the elbow.

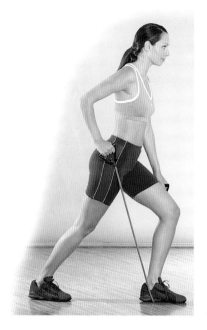
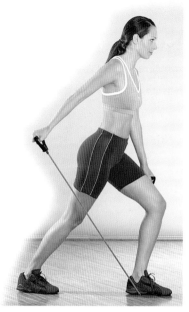

- In reverse, the forearm is moved back to the starting position so that the tube still offers some resistance.

Advice:

- Avoid moving your pelvis or shoulder girdle. During the exercise the range of motion of your hand is rather small; only your forearm is in motion.
- Hold your head as a natural extension of the spine.
- The tighter you keep the tubing on the side of the active arm, the greater the impact will be on your muscles.

Strength Training for Your Shoulders

Stiffness in the neck and shoulders is extremely common and often causes headaches. For this reason you should train your shoulders with care. During these exercises the shoulders will be trained simultaneously with other body parts. If you suffer from a stiff neck and shoulders, focus on stretching first.

Side Arm Raises

- Stand in walking position and keep your back in line with your right leg, which is extended backward.
- With your front leg stand in the middle of the rubber tube.
- Hold the handles so that the back of your hands are facing sideways.
- Lift up your right arm so that it is almost extended to your shoulder.
- Return to the starting position.
- Be sure to work both sides. The tube should always keep a basic resistance and never sag.
- This exercise trains the front and midsection of your shoulder muscles.

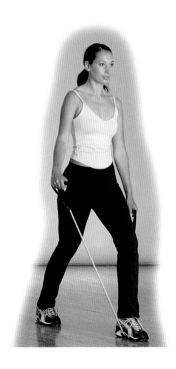
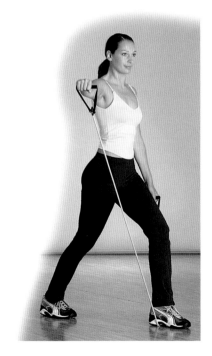

Info

Variation A with a hand weight can also be performed sitting. Make sure to keep your back straight and upright during the entire exercise.

Tip

To add variation, you may lift both arms simultaneously. Always keep your wrists in neutral position.

Info

How your torso is positioned is extremely important. Always keep your body straight and pull your shoulders down during the exercise. Do not lean back.

Variation A

As an alternative to exercise handles, you can use a hand weight.

Variation B

- This variation is the same as Side Arm Raises on page 44, except that you lift up your almost-extended arms in front of your body (no photograph).

- Remember: do not lift your arms higher than your shoulders.
- This exercise mainly works the front section of your shoulder muscles.

Variation C

Variation B can also be performed with hand weights in a seated position.

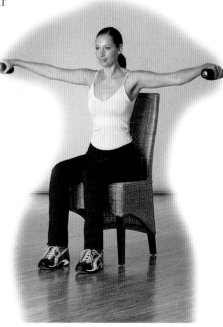

45

Standing Row

- Stand in a walking position and secure the middle of the tube with your front foot. Both knees are slightly bent. Place the handles on top of each other and hold them with both hands. The back of your hands should face away from your body and the wrists should be kept straight.

- Pull the tube close to your body and up to your chest. During this exercise your elbows should reach high. Keep your shoulders pulled down at all times. Your torso should form one line with the extended back leg. The tube should always provide minimal resistance.

Variations

- To add a challenge, stand on the tube with both legs.
- You can also use hand weights with this exercise. Take one weight in each hand and bring them together.

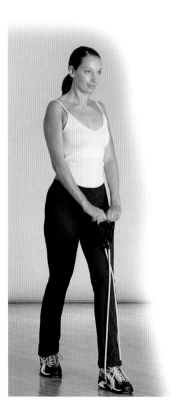
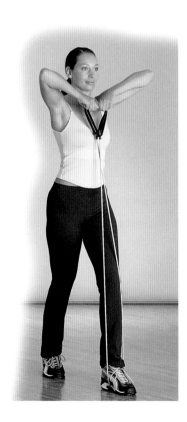

Pullbacks

- Sit down. Rest your feet on your heels and keep your legs hip-width apart with your knees slightly bent.
- Place the tube around your soles. Grab the handles so that the back of your hands face backward.

- Stabilize your back and keep your torso upright. Keep your shoulders pulled down.
- Move your slightly extended arms back while you pull your shoulder blades together downward and straighten your chest forward.

Variation

- Grab the tube with palms facing backward. Keep your wrists stabilized to avoid unnecessary pressure on the forearm muscles.

Info

With this exercise you also train your back muscles and triceps.

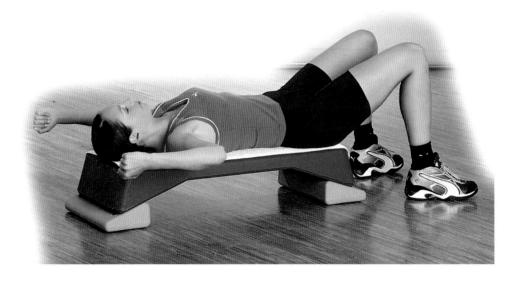

Strength Training for Your Chest

Often the chest muscles, or pectorals, are trained with special intensity. Remember to strengthen the upper back muscles that are parallel to your pectorals in order to improve your posture. One of the following exercises that we specifically recommend is the push-up (page 51). Very few exercises are as compact and effective as push-ups, yet at the same time as unpopular due to their degree of difficulty. With push-ups you not only train your chest muscles but also your shoulders and triceps.

Butterfly with Arms Bent

- Lie down on your back, preferably on a step. Keep your knees bent with your feet flat on the floor. Deliberately pull your navel toward your spine. Position your arms next to your head. Bend the forearms in a right angle to your upper arms.
- Exhale while moving your

bent arms together in front of your torso.

- Afterward, open your arms and inhale.
- Always make sure that your upper arms and forearms form a right angle. To perform the exercise effectively, you should always hold your arms parallel to the floor in the starting position to maintain a minimal level of tension in your pectorals.

Variation

To increase the intensity of this exercise use hand weights.

Info

Although in the beginning you work without hand weights, this exercise is still quite strenuous, because you are working against gravity.

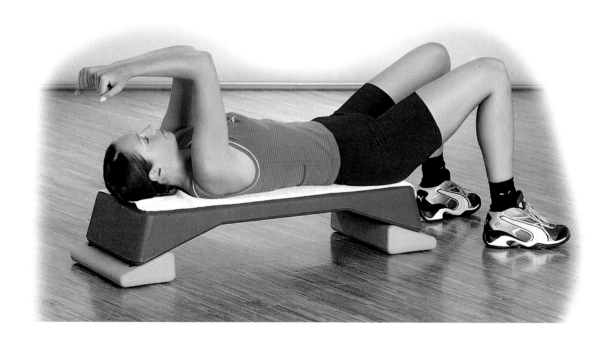

Bench Press

- This exercise can be performed best with hand weights and lying on a step. Lay your head and back on the step. Keep your knees bent with your feet flat on the floor.
- Lift your bent arms straight up. Keep your shoulders pulled toward your buttocks during the exercise. Wrists remain in neutral position.
- Perform this exercise slowly and with concentration.

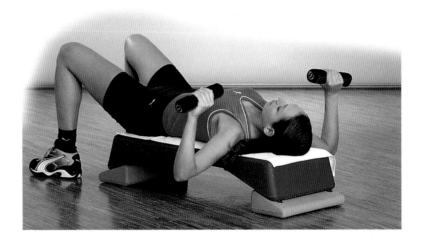

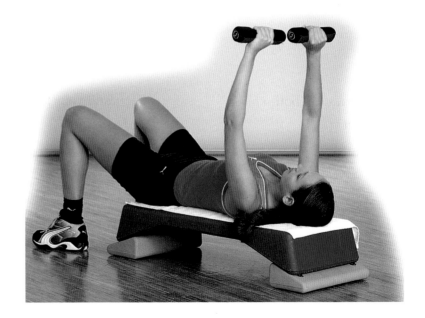

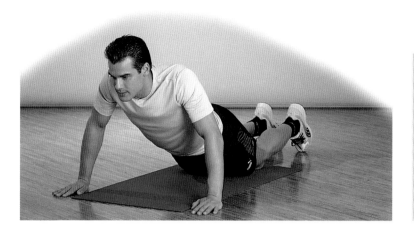

Tip

During the exercise make sure to always breathe evenly: inhale when relaxing your muscles and exhale when tightening them.

Push-ups

- Start on all fours with your arms positioned relatively wide apart and at the same level with your head. Your weight should rest mainly on your torso. Your legs should rest on both knees and feet.
- Support your back by tightening your abs.
- Bend your arms and move your torso toward the floor.
- Afterward, extend your arms again and lift yourself up.

- Remember not to overstretch your elbows.

Variation

- A more complicated variation is a push-up with your legs extended and slightly apart and your feet resting on your toes.
- During the exercise do not allow the body to go lax, but preserve some tension. With this extremely effective exercise you also train your shoulder muscles and triceps.

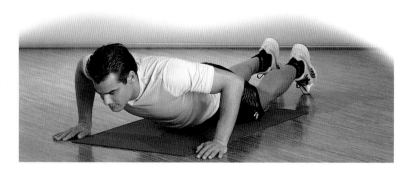

Strength Training for Your Upper Back

Interestingly, the back muscles do not start with the shoulders, but rather the muscles around the cervical spine. Did you know that our cervical vertebrae actually have to carry a weight of about 17 pounds (8 kilograms)? That is how much our head weighs on top of the small cervical vertebrae. The following exercises are performed partly statically and partly dynamically. Static strength training consists of exercises that are performed without movement. Dynamic exercises are, by contrast, those that are performed in motion. Perform all exercises for the upper back slowly, fluidly, and with strength.

Neck and Throat (Static)

- Sit down on a chair and push your buttocks directly up against the back of the chair. Keep your torso upright and your shoulder blades pulled toward your buttocks.
- Fold your hands behind your back and keep your elbows facing sideways.
- Press the back of your head against your palms. Your hands are putting pressure on the back of your head.
- Place your hands on your forehead. Apply pressure

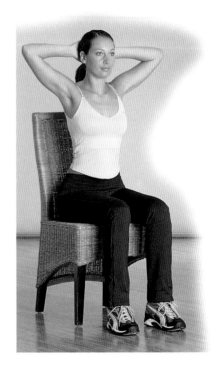

to your head and counterpressure to your hands.

Variation

- To strengthen your cervical muscles, place the left ball

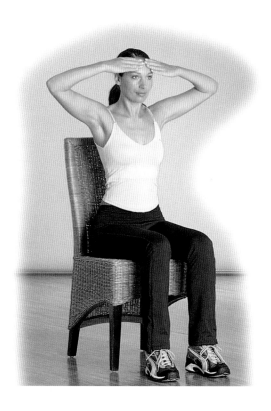

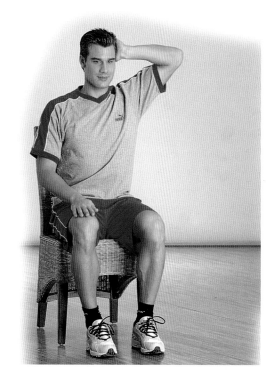

of your thumb above your left ear. Your elbow points to the side.

- Apply pressure and counterpressure. Remember to keep your shoulders pulled down during the entire exercise.
- Hold the position for 10–30 seconds each time.
- Do not forget to switch arms.

Info

During these exercises always hold your head in a neutral, straight, and upright position and do not lean to the side.

Sitting Row (Dynamic)

■ Take the Thera-Band or exercise handle in both hands and sit down on the floor.

■ Wrap the tube around your feet as shown in the picture.

■ Your legs should be shoulder-width apart; knees slightly bent.

■ Lift your torso up and

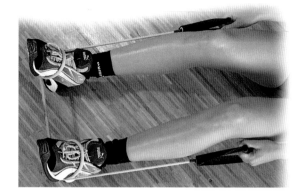

keep your chest facing forward. Look straight ahead. Keep your head straight to avoid straining your neck. Keep your arms close to your body.

■ Pull your elbows back to

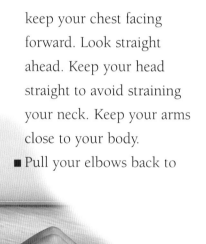

Info

This exercise is especially challenging because it requires a great deal of strength from your entire back.

your sides. Make sure that you deliberately pull your shoulder blades down toward your spine.

■ Move back to the starting position. The tube should

offer slight resistance even in the starting position.

Variation

■ Wrap the middle of the tube around the soles of your feet so that the handles are positioned on the sides. Then cross the tube in front of your body. Hold your elbows at shoulder level, with your shoulders pulled back at all times. The back of your hands face the ceiling and your wrists are straight.

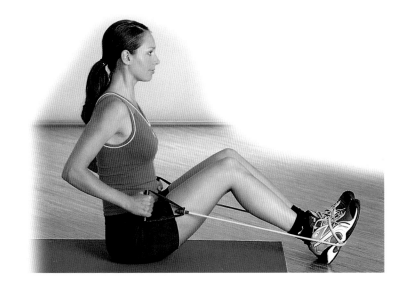

■ Lift your elbows up to your shoulders and then, with control, move them back to the starting position.

Tip

To increase resistance, open your legs more—the tube is shortened and the exercise becomes more difficult.

Lat Pull Down (Dynamic)

- Stand upright with your legs shoulder-width apart.
- Wrap the tube around your hands so that a loop is formed on both sides. Place the tube over your head.
- Holding the tube tightly, pull it down behind your head. The tube is positioned close to your body and your shoulder blades are pulled together.
- Slowly move back to the starting position. During the entire exercise, keep your wrists straight, elbows slightly bent, and head erect.

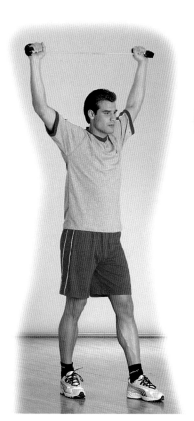

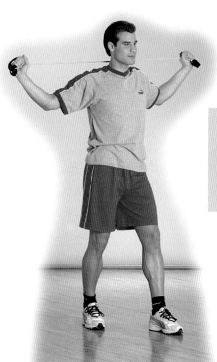

Tip

Tighten your abs and glutes to avoid a hollow back.

Variation

- You can also perform this exercise lying on your stomach. Open your legs shoulder-width apart, with your toes touching the floor.

- Tighten your abs and glutes during the variation. To avoid unnecessary swaying, palce a rolled-up towel under your hips.

- This exercise and its variant can also be performed with one arm. Make sure that the tubing remains tight at all times.

- With this exercise you also train your shoulder muscles.

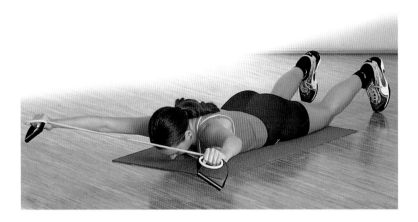

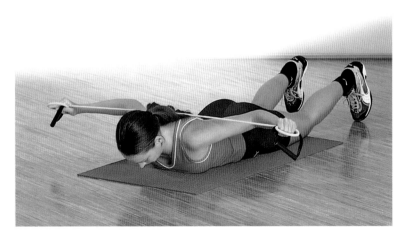

External Rotation (Dynamic)

- Stand upright with your legs shoulder-width apart and knees slightly bent, your palms facing inward.
- Wrap the Thera-Band or exercise handle tube around the back of your hands and between your thumb and index fingers. Your upper arm and forearm should form a 90-degree angle.
- Hold the tube tight and move your forearms against this resistance to the sides. The elbows remain close to the body.
- Slowly move back to the starting position and make sure that the tube is kept tight at all times.

Variation

- Perform the movement slowly several times with only your right hand and then a few times with only your left hand.

Info

Push your chest bone forward and slightly tighten your abs and glutes to better stabilize your body.

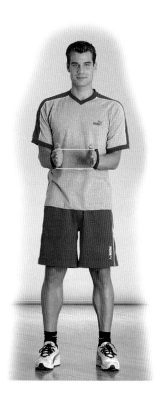

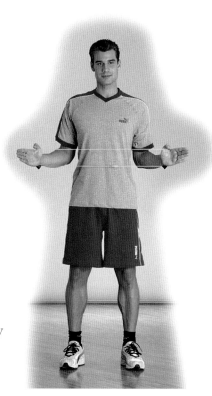

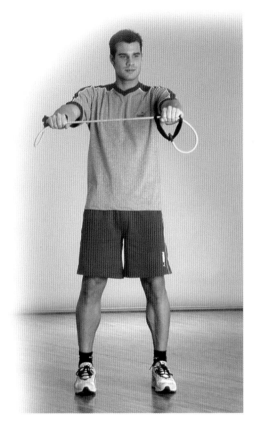 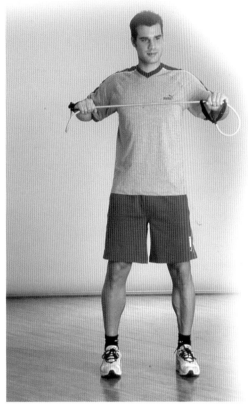

Butterfly Inverse (Dynamic)

- Stand with your legs hip-width apart and hold the exercise handle in front of your chest with each hand holding a handle.
- Wrap the tube around your hands until you feel resistance.
- Flex your arms and, with your elbows forward, move them toward your body.
- Move your arms back to the front.

Side Arm Raises (Dynamic)

- Start on all fours with your left hand resting on the mat. Hold a hand weight in your right hand. Your left arm is almost extended and slightly bent at the elbow.

- Support your back by tightening your abs. Look to the floor so that your head forms a straight line with your back.

- Lift your right arm sideways up to your shoulders and then move it back again.

- Hold the hand weight in neutral position—as a straight extension of your forearm. Do not forget to switch arms.

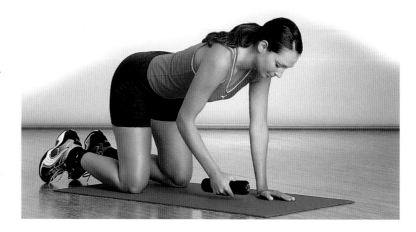

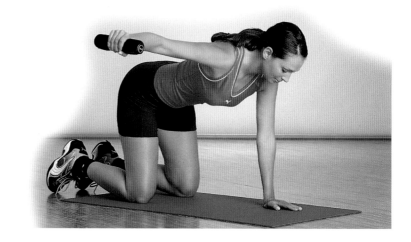

Info

Hold the supporting arm slightly bent at all times to avoid unnecessary pressure on your elbows and shoulders.

Elbow Raises (Dynamic)

- Lie on your stomach. Open your legs shoulder-width apart with your feet resting on your toes. Slightly tighten your buttocks.

- In this starting position fold your hands at head level, the lower hand touching the floor. Rest your forehead on the back of your hands with your elbows pointing outward.

- Always keeping contact between your upper body, your lower hand, and the floor, slowly lift up your elbows.

- Make sure to pull your shoulders toward your buttocks during the exercise and pull your shoulder blades together while lifting your elbows.

- Afterward, slowly lower your elbows, but do not let them touch the floor.

Tip

To support your lumbar spine we recommend placing a rolled-up towel under your hips.

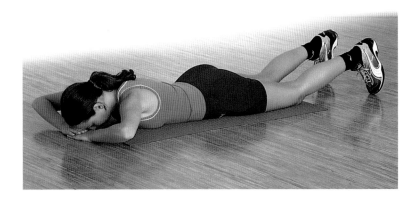

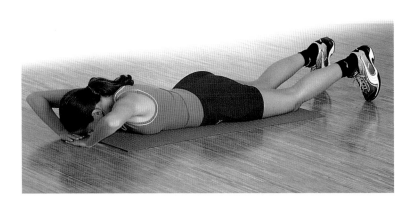

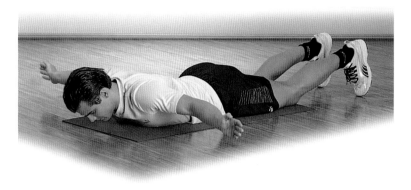

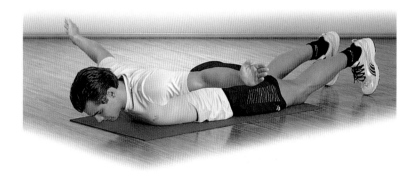

head should form a straight extension of your spine, which means you look to the floor.

- Slowly lift up your slightly extended arms through your shoulder blades.

- Afterward, slowly move your arms back to the starting position. Your thumbs are still pointing up. Make sure that your hands do not touch the floor and keep a minimal tension in your back muscles.

Arm Raises Facing Down (Dynamic)

- Use the same starting position for Elbow Raises on page 61. Extend your arms sideways and keep your elbows slightly bent. Point your thumbs toward the ceiling. Your torso should remain comfortably on the floor during the entire exercise and your

Variation

- To increase the intensity of this exercise we recommend using hand weights.

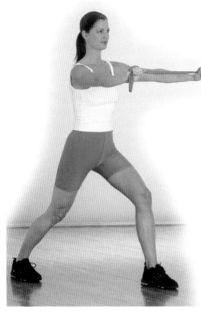

Back Pull (Dynamic)

■ The following exercise focuses on the muscles between your shoulder blades. These muscles are important for straight posture. When strong, these muscles prevent a hunched-over back. It is very important that these muscle groups be trained regularly.

■ Stand in a lunge position and hold the Thera-Band with both hands.

■ Slowly bend your front leg.

■ Extend your arms in front of you and stretch the band to the side. Exhale deeply. The movement is complete once both arms are extended sideways.

■ During the exercise make sure to keep a straight posture. Do not pull up your shoulders. Keep your head as an extension to your spine by pulling your chin toward your chest, thus forming a kind of double chin. Make sure that the band is always tight.

■ You should feel a direct impact on your upper back muscles and an indirect impact on your upper thighs and buttocks. These muscle groups are necessary for correct posture.

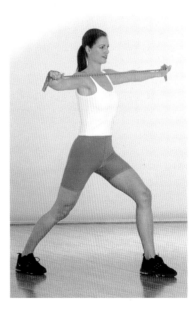

Strength Training for Your Lower Back

Many people experience lower back pain. For this reason a systematic training is very important, even though the exercises for the lower back are rather strenuous. Only through a balanced training of the lower and upper back can you provide your spine with the necessary stability. In contrast to strength training for other muscle groups, where breathing should be coordinated with the movement, we recommend that you breathe slowly and evenly during these exercises. Otherwise, you can easily stiffen your spine and form the condition known as swayback.

Lifting Torso Facedown (Dynamic)

- Lie facedown and build up minimal tension by opening your legs shoulder-width apart and resting your feet on your toes.

- Tighten your glutes. Keep looking down—this guarantees that your spine is held as an extension of the body. Your palms lie on your buttocks.

- Lift your head and shoulders simultaneously.

- Afterward, lower your head and shoulders. Avoid touching the floor in order to keep a basic tension in your back muscles.

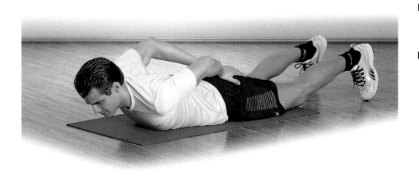

Variations

- To make this exercise even more intense, lift up your torso so that your chest moves slowly off the ground. Always remember to maintain your head as if it were a straight extension of your body.

- Changing the position of your arm will increase the level of difficulty even more. Place your arms over one another and point your elbows outward. Your forehead rests on the back of your hands. The movements are the same as above.

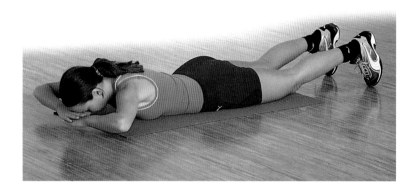

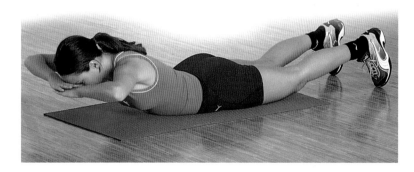

Tips

If you tend to sway, we recommend placing a rolled-up towel under your pelvis. This will support your lumbar spine.

During the exercise always make sure to keep your legs and the tips of your toes on the ground.

Leg Raises Facedown (Dynamic)

- Lie on your stomach and bend your arms so that you can rest your forehead on the back of your hands.
- With your feet resting on your toes, tighten your glutes.
- Slowly lift up the right, slightly extended leg while your left knee remains on the floor.
- Lower your right leg without touching the floor. During the exercise your torso and hips should remain on the floor at all times.
- Do not forget to alternate your legs and perform an equal number of repetitions with your left leg.

Info

With this exercise you will also train your glutes.

Variation

- To make the exercise more intense, extend your left arm in front of you.
- Slowly lift your left arm and your right leg a few inches (a couple of centimeters) off the floor and then lower your arm and leg again. Avoid touching the floor with your active leg and arm.
- Do not forget to switch arms and legs.

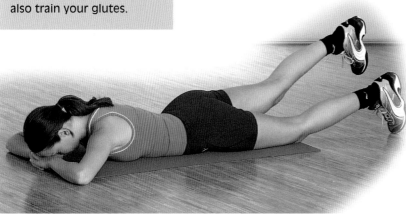

Back Extension Facedown (Dynamic)

- Lie on your stomach and build up a minimal amount of tension by opening your legs shoulder-width apart and resting your feet on your toes. Maintain this minimal tension throughout the entire exercise.

- Extend your arms to the front. During this strengthening exercise it is especially important to pull your arms and legs forward and not lift up your torso.

- Once you slowly release the tension, your arms and legs should not touch the floor. This ensures that a minimal amount of tension in your back muscles is maintained.

Variation

- If you are more advanced and your back muscles are well trained, you may use hand weights to increase the intensity of the exercise.

Info

This exercise is especially strenuous, because of the wide arm movements, and demands a high degree of strength. Make sure to perform the exercise smoothly.

67

Pull In Walking Position (Dynamic)

- Stand in walking position and move the Thera-Band underneath your front leg. Hold the loose ends.
- Move your arms in front of your chest. The band should be kept tight.
- Bend your straight torso a little to the front. Inhale deeply. Remember to keep a straight posture!
- Straighten up against the resistance of the band. Exhale deeply.

- After some repetitions you will feel an increased blood flow in your back extensor.

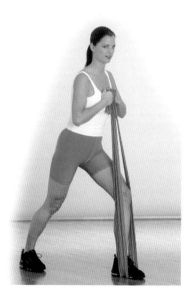

Tip

After you feel comfortable with this exercise, change your starting position. Lift up your rear leg and perform the exercise again. It will feel more intense. Remember to keep your posture. These exercises will strengthen your entire back.

Oblique Pulls (Dynamic)

- Lie face down on the step bench so that your hip is positioned on the edge of the bench. The knee and tip of the toe of your right leg should touch the floor. Extend your left leg. Place your left forearm on the floor and extend your right arm in front of you. Keep eyes on the floor.

- Simultaneously lift up your right arm and left leg.

- Breathe evenly and do not forget to switch sides.

Variation

- It is also possible to perform the oblique pull on the floor without a step.

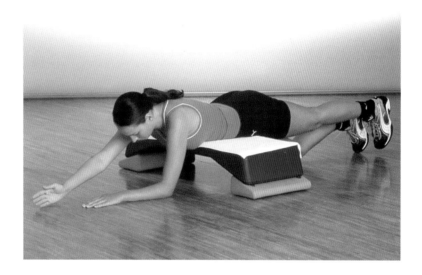

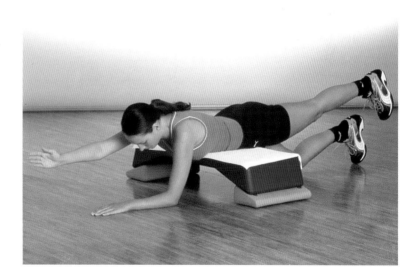

Strength Training for Your Stomach

The abdominals consist of four different muscles: the rectus abdominis, the two obliques, and the deeper transversus abdominis muscle. Regular training of the abs provides excellent protection against back problems.

Rectus Abdominis Exercises

Basic Crunches

- Lie on your back with your feet almost forming a right angle. To deactivate the hip extensors, touch the floor with only your heels.
- Your lumbar spine remains firmly on the floor during this exercise.
- Slightly lift up your torso while slightly rounding your back. Pull both arms sideways to the front. Face your palms toward the ceiling.
- Lift your torso only with your abs, not with the help of your arms.
- Move back to the starting position.

Info

- Make sure that your body forms an extension of your torso. Your chin should be positioned about a hand's width apart from your chest and your eyes should face the ceiling.
- To avoid a hollow back, pull your navel toward the floor at all times.
- Be aware that the tension experienced during this exercise originates in the abs.
- Perform the exercise slowly and without momentum.
- Breathe evenly: inhale when you lift yourself up and pull your navel toward your spine so that you bring your lower ribs to your hips. Exhale once your body is lowered.
- Try to keep the shoulder blades off the ground during the lowering movement in order to keep a minimal amount of tension within your muscles to achieve an ideal strengthening effect.

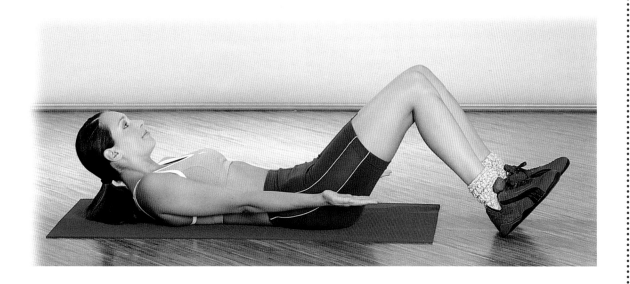

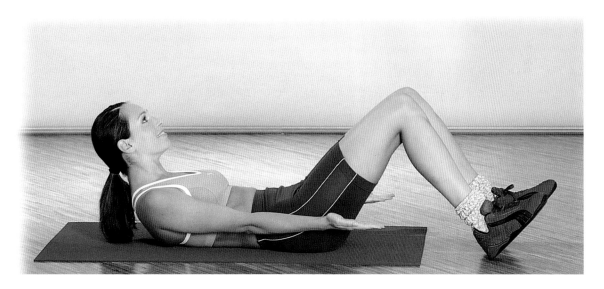

Variation A

- Perform this exercise the same as in Basic Crunches on page 70.
- In addition, cross both arms over your chest. Do not push your shoulders forward.

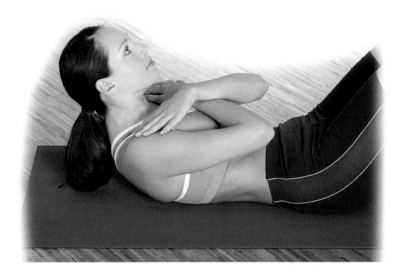

Variation B

- Perform this exercise the same as in Variation A.
- In addition, use hand weights to intensify the exercise.

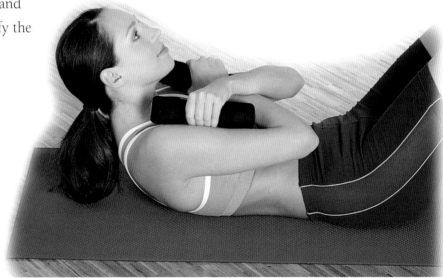

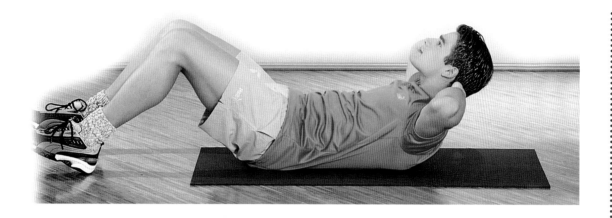

Variation C

■ Perform this exercise the same as in Basic Crunches on page 70.

■ Support your neck with both hands and hold your elbows outward during the entire exercise. Fix a point on the ceiling with your eyes.

■ Deliberately work with your abs and do not push your head up with your hands!

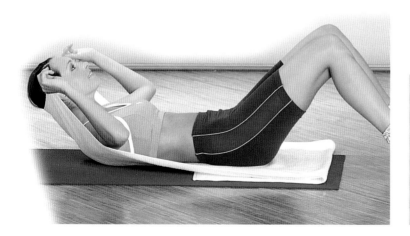

Tip

You can also perform this exercise with a towel, grabbing a corner with each hand.

Variation D

■ Perform this exercise the same as in Basic Crunches on page 70.

■ Extend your arms over your head. Keep your head between your arms during the entire exercise.

■ To increase the level of difficulty, use hand weights.

■ Perform the basic crunches and their variations in 2–3 sets with 15–20 repetitions, depending on your fitness level.

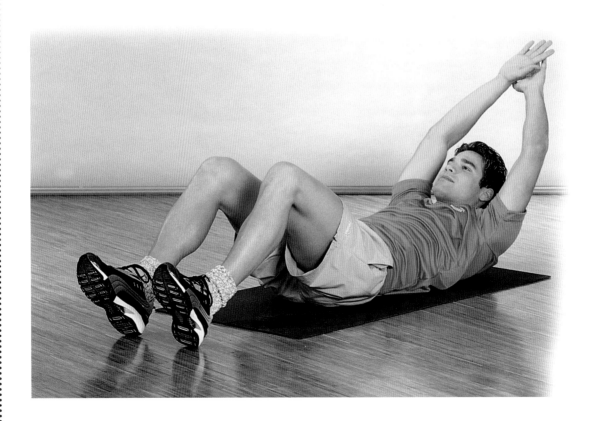

Reverse Crunches

- Lie on your back with both legs bent and lifted.
- Let your feet dangle and cross your arms behind your head.
- Slowly move your hips tightly toward your lower ribs. Afterward, slightly release the tension and do not touch the floor anymore with your hips. Your head, arms, and torso touch the floor at all times.
- Depending on your fitness level, perform 2–3 sets with 15–20 repetitions.

Tip

Deliberately exhale while curling up.

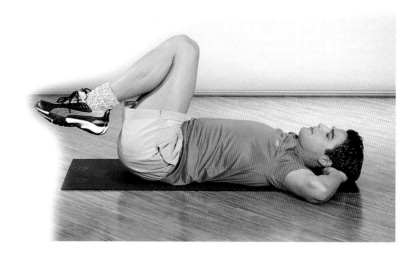

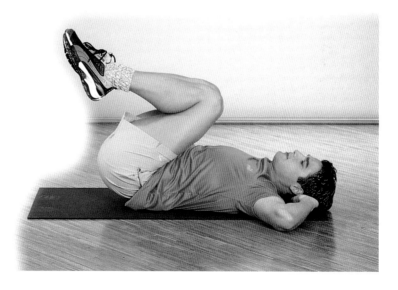

Your range of motion does not have to be very wide. What is important is that you feel the tension in your abs, which you control by placing a palm on your stomach during the exercise.

Pelvis Tilt

- Lie on your back and extend your slightly bent legs to the ceiling. The tips of your toes are pulled toward your knees. The back of your head rests on your palms.
- Lift your buttocks off the floor without momentum and lift your legs up straight; then slowly lower them.

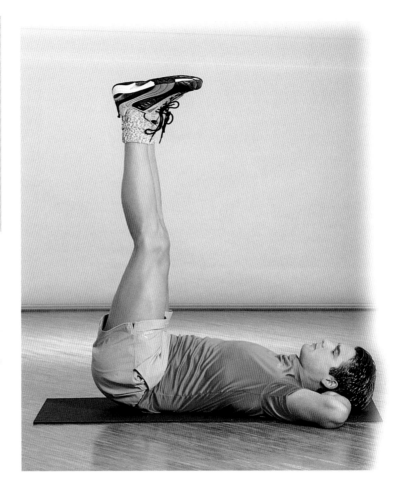

- Shortly before reaching the floor, lift up your buttocks again.

- Make sure that your head, arms, and torso touch the floor during the entire exercise.

■ Even if this is especially difficult, continue to breathe consciously and avoid pressure breathing or holding your breath.

Variation

■ Use a Thera-Band or exercise handle to make this exercise more difficult. Wrap the tube around the middle of your soles to ensure it will not slip off. During the exercise the tube should not sag and has to be kept slightly tight.

■ Your extended arms lie next to your body and your palms face the floor.

■ Depending on your fitness level, perform 2–3 sets with 15–20 repetitions.

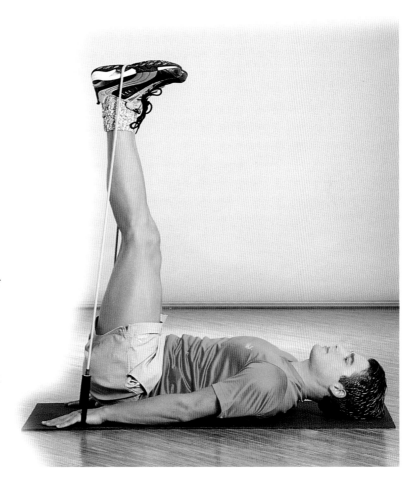

Info

Consciously work with your abs and do not use your hands to push yourself up.

Oblique Exercises

Oblique Crunches

- Lie on your back with your left leg bent and resting on the heel.
- Place your right foot on your left upper thigh while slightly turning your right knee outward.
- Your right arm lies extended on the floor.
- With your left arm extended, move it diagonally across your right upper thigh. Lift up your torso diagonally.
- Move back to the starting position, but keep your left shoulder blade off the floor at all times. Make sure to keep your head in a neutral position during the entire exercise.

Variation A

- Use the same starting position as in Oblique Crunches, but support your neck with your left palm while your elbow is pointing to the side.

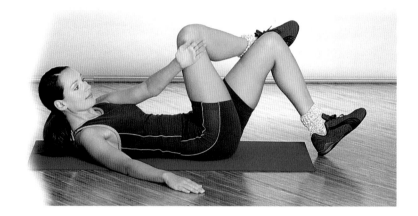

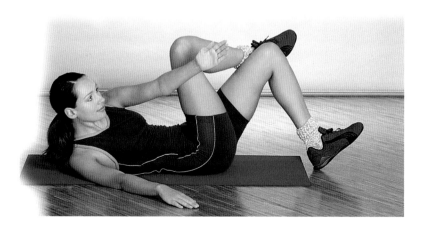

■ With your left shoulder
  move diagonally toward
  your right knee.

Variation B

■ Use the same starting
  position as in Oblique
  Crunches on page 78, but
  rest both legs on the floor.

■ Let both your knees fall to
  the right side. Your hands
  support the back of your
  head.

■ Slowly lift your torso off
  the floor. When lowering

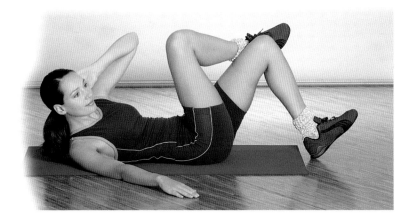

your torso, avoid touching
the floor as much as
possible.

■ Perform 2–3 sets with
  15–20 repetitions per side.

Tip

Variation B becomes easier if
you cross both arms over
your chest. Do not forget to
switch sides.

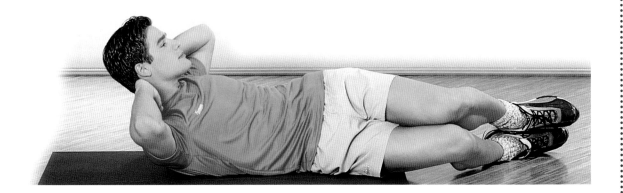

Side Crunches

- Start by lying on one side. Legs rest, slightly bent, on top of each other.
- Stabilize your body by placing your left forearm on the floor and placing your right hand at chest level in front of you. Your head should not "sink" below your shoulders.
- Lift your pelvis and legs off the floor until your spine is straight.
- Move your pelvis and legs back again; avoid touching the floor.

Variation A

- Perform the same routine as in Side Crunches, but extend your legs completely on the floor.

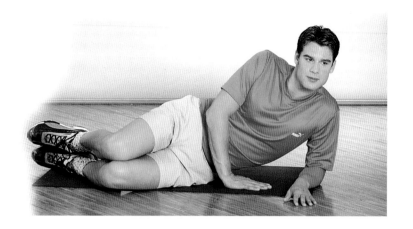

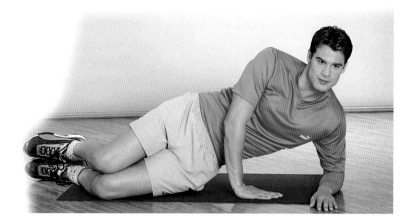

Tip

If the exercise is too hard for you in the beginning, push up your torso slightly with your right supporting arm.

Variation B

■ Perform the same routine as in Side Crunches on page 80, but place your right arm on your right upper thigh.

■ Perform 2–3 sets with 15–20 repetitions per side.

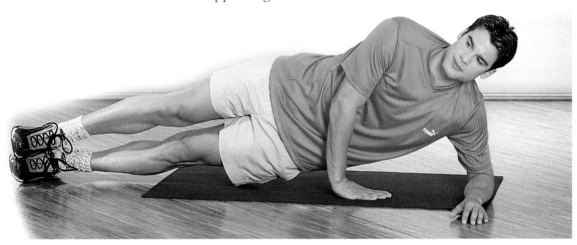

Info

Make sure not to fall backward.

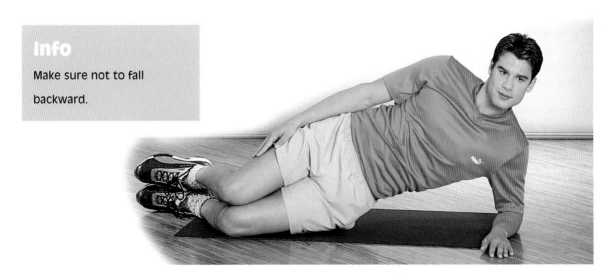

Thera-Band Crunches

- Lie on your back and bend both knees. Your upper and lower thighs should form a 90-degree angle.
- Pull the tips of your toes toward your face and place the band under your feet. Make sure the band fits tightly. Take the loose ends of the band in both hands.
- Lift up your head and shoulders while

simultaneously pulling the band with both hands. The execution of this exercise is similar to a rowing movement.

- Keep an eye on your posture. Do not curl your body; lift your torso up straight. Fix your eyes on the ceiling.
- Inhale when lifting up and exhale when lowering your torso.
- Hint: Perform this exercise slowly and without momentum.

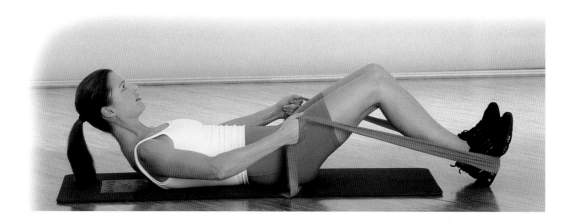

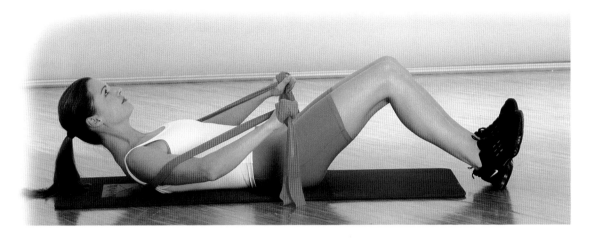

Variation

- Lie on your back and bend your knees.
- Place the Thera-Band under your shoulders and take the loose ends in your hands.
- Hold your arms slightly bent in front of you.
- Lift up your torso while slightly moving to your right. Extend your left arm and stretch the band. You will feel a slight pressure on your obliques. This exercise will also train your pectorals as you stretch your arms against the resistance of the Thera-Band.
- Exhale while holding the tension; then inhale and lower your torso again.
- Perform the exercise on the other side.

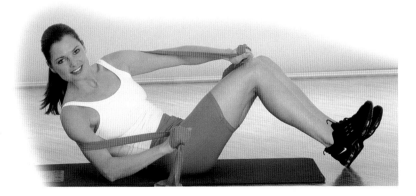

Total Body Stabilization

Exercise 1

- Start on all fours. Extend your left leg backward and your right arm in front of you.
- Stabilize your back by pulling your stomach in slightly. Keep breathing naturally.
- The elbow of your supporting arm is slightly bent. You should form a straight line from your right hand to your left leg.
- Remain in this position for about 10–30 seconds and then switch sides.

Info

The tighter your body, the easier it will be to keep your balance.

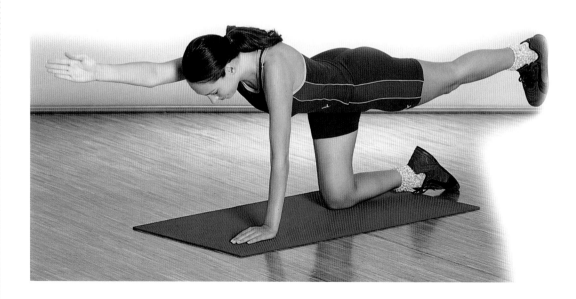

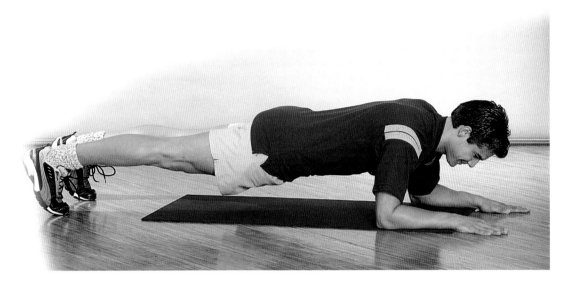

Exercise 2

- Support yourself with your forearms. Keep your legs shoulder-width apart and rest on your toes.

- Pull your shoulder blades toward your buttocks with your eyes facing the floor so that your head forms an extension of your spine.

- Hold your body tight and make sure your back is straight. Your body should be tight as a board.

- Breathe calmly and evenly and do not hold your breath.

- Remain in this position for about 10–30 seconds.

Info

This exercise is especially strenuous and requires a high degree of tension in your whole body. Ideally, you should perform it in front of a mirror in order to know whether or not you are really forming a straight line with your body.

Strength Training for Your Buttocks

Reclining Leg Lifts

- Lie on one side with your lower leg slightly bent and your upper leg almost extended. The tips of the toes of your upper leg are pulled toward your shin.
- Position your pelvis so that your hips lie parallel on top of each other.
- Your upper arm is supported by your hand in front of your chest to stabilize your torso. Your head lies on your lower arm.

- Lift your upper leg until your foot is positioned slightly above your hip.
- Lower your leg again without touching the lower leg.

- Do not forget to switch legs.

Variation

- In order to intensify your workout, you can either wrap a Thera-Band around

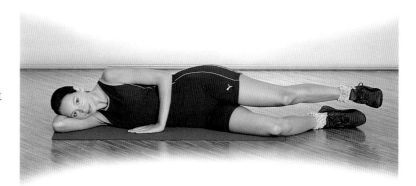

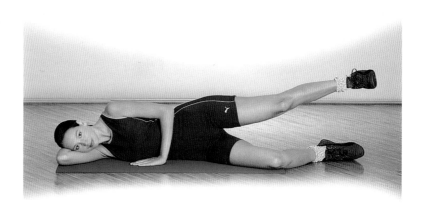

your ankles or exercise with a hand weight on top of your upper leg.

- With the leg raise you also train your outer leg muscles.
- Perform 2–3 sets with 15–20 repetitions per leg.

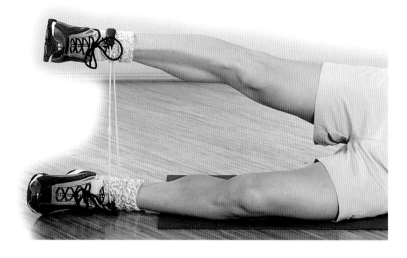

Info

The closer the weights are to your knee, the higher the resistance is. The closer the weights are to your hip, the easier the exercise is. The placement of the weights allows you to choose the level of difficulty according to your own personal fitness level.

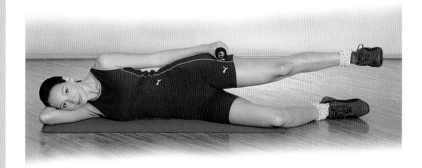

Standing Leg Lift

- Stand upright in front or next to a chair with your legs shoulder-width apart. Hold on to the back of the chair.
- During this exercise your torso should remain upright and your shoulders pulled slightly back toward your buttocks.
- Both knees are slightly bent and your abs are slightly tightened.
- Balance your weight on your right leg and move your left leg to the side while keeping your torso straight.
- Move your leg back to its starting position, without allowing your foot to touch the floor.
- Do not forget to switch legs per side.

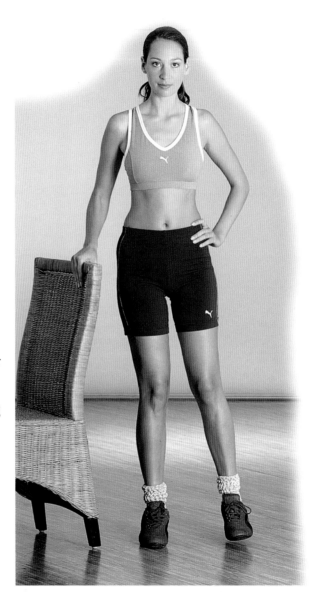

Variation

■ Advanced exercisers may increase the intensity of this exercise with the help of a Thera-Band.

■ Perform 2–3 sets with 15–20 repetitions.

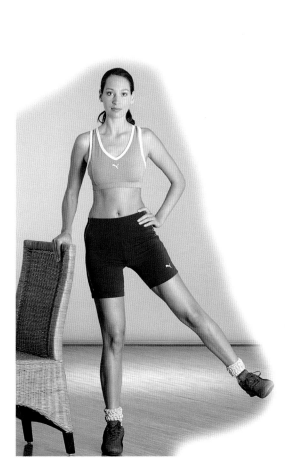

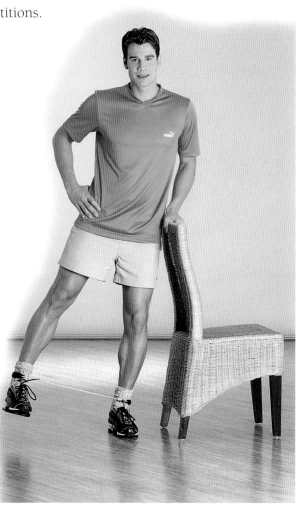

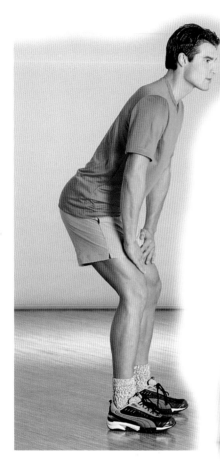

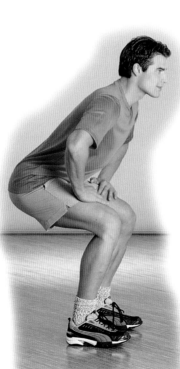

Narrow Squat

- Stand with legs shoulder-width apart and knees slightly bent. Support your torso by resting your hands on your upper thighs while keeping your back straight and firm.
- Push your buttocks back and down, as if sitting in a chair. Do not push your knees forward. During the entire exercise your body weight rests solely on your heels and your torso should be kept as upright as possible.
- Move back into the starting position.

Tip

In case you have difficulty keeping your balance, use a chair for support.

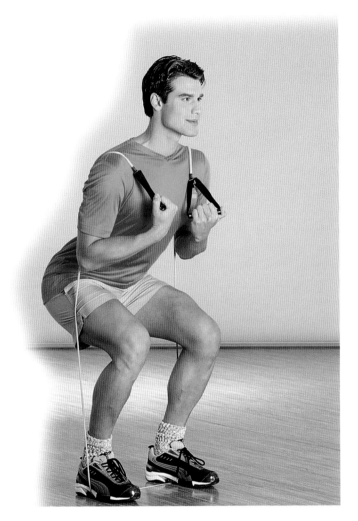

Variation

- With both feet stand in the middle of an exercise handle and pull the handles over your shoulders.
- To put as little strain on your wrists as possible, make sure that the back of your hands face away from your body.
- You should perform this variation only if you feel secure and only when you are familiar with the basic exercise.
- This exercise trains the front and rear leg muscles as well.
- Perform 2–3 sets with 15–20 repetitions.

Tip

Placing a towel around your shoulders will protect you from possible bruises from the exercise handle.

Asymmetrical Squat

- For this exercise you will need a step bench.
- Stand with legs shoulder width apart as close as possible to the step and place your right foot on it.
- Keep your back straight and move your buttocks back and down. Pay attention to your knees, as they should not be pushed upward. You weight should rest on the heel of your standing leg.
- To help you keep your balance, move your extended arms forward while lowering your buttocks.
- Move back to the starting position.
- Do not forget to switch legs.

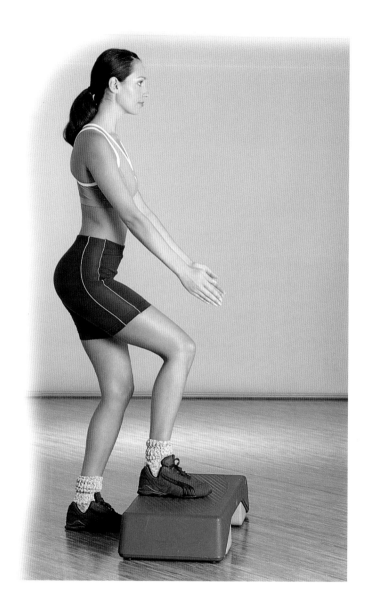

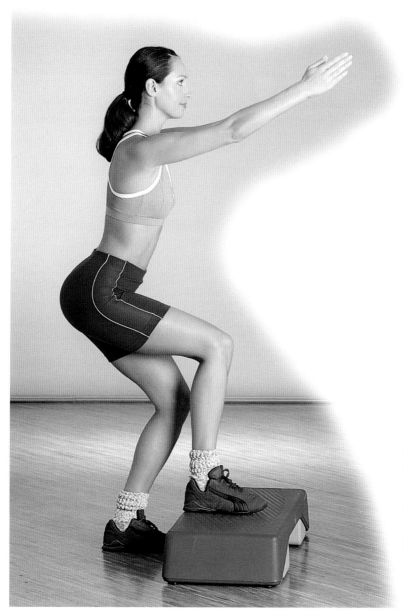

- This exercise trains the anterior and posterior leg muscles as well.
- Perform 2–3 sets with 15–20 repetitions per leg.

Tip

As an alternative to the step bench, you can use a 8-inch (20-centimeter)-high firm box or a foot bench for this exercise.

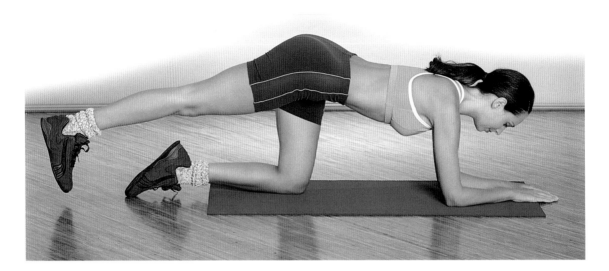

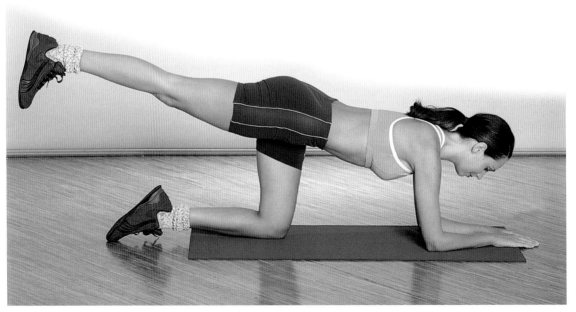

Straight Leg Raise on All Fours

- Start on all fours while supporting your torso with your forearms. Your shoulder and elbow joints, as well as your hip and knee joints, form a straight line.
- During the entire exercise keep your back straight and keep your head as an extension of your spine while you face the floor.
- Extend one leg backward and lift it up until it forms a straight line with your body. Do not move your hip up.
- Move back to the starting position while the toes of your extended leg do not touch the floor. Do not forget to switch legs.

Variation

- Use an exercise handle to increase resistance.
- With this exercise you will also train your lower back muscles.

- 2–3 sets with 15–20 repetitions per leg, depending on your fitness level.

Tip

Slightly tighten your abs to really keep your back straight.

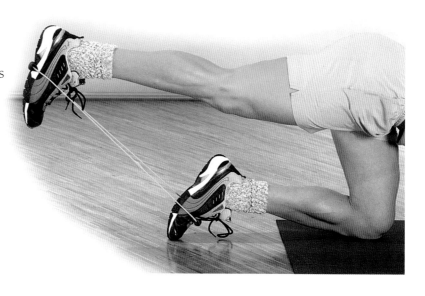

Bent Leg Lift on All Fours

- Start on all fours, with your torso resting on your forearms. Your shoulder and elbow joints and your hip and knee joints form a straight line.

- Keep your back straight during the entire exercise, with your head as an extension of your spine and your eyes facing the floor. Both shoulder blades are pulled toward your buttocks.

- Start with your right bent leg and keep the knee a few inches (centimeters) off the floor.

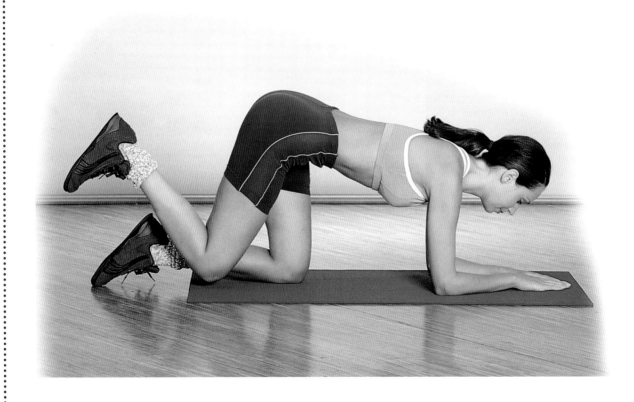

- Avoid swaying.
- Using strength, push the heel of your bent leg toward the ceiling. The angle of your knee remains the same. Once the knee and hip joints form a straight line you have reached your final position. During this exercise you should be careful not to lean back with your hip. Only move the active leg.
- Move back to the starting position without allowing the knee of the active leg to touch the floor.
- Do not forget to switch legs.

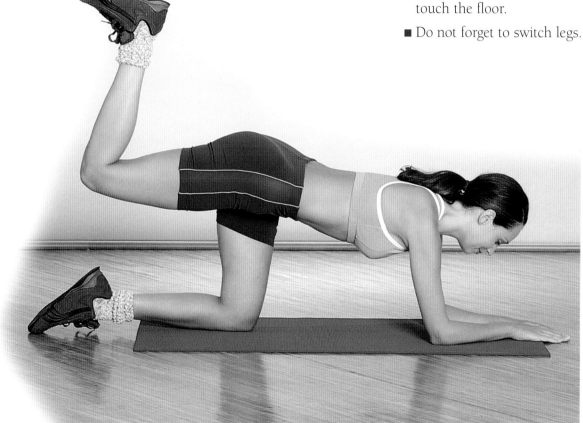

Variation A

■ Use the exercise handle to increase resistance. Make sure that the cord is positioned in the middle of the sole of the active foot.

■ In order to keep your balance during this exercise, your weight should be balanced equally on your leg and forearms. Avoid resting your weight on your bent leg.

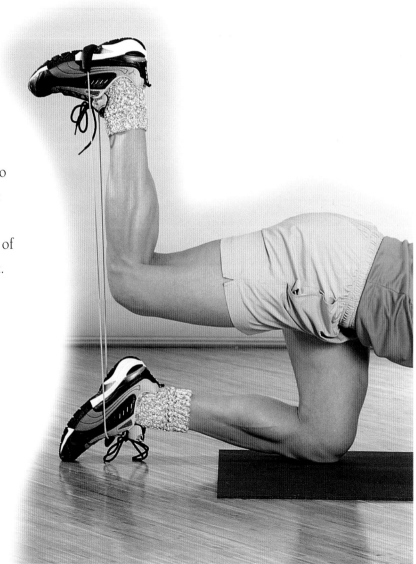

Variation B

- Place a hand weight in the hollow of the knee of the active leg.
- With this exercise you also train your back muscles and the posterior upper thigh muscles.
- Perform 2–3 sets with 15–20 repetitions, depending on your fitness level.

Info

Always lift your leg just up to your hip joints; otherwise you might unnecessarily strain your back through swaying.

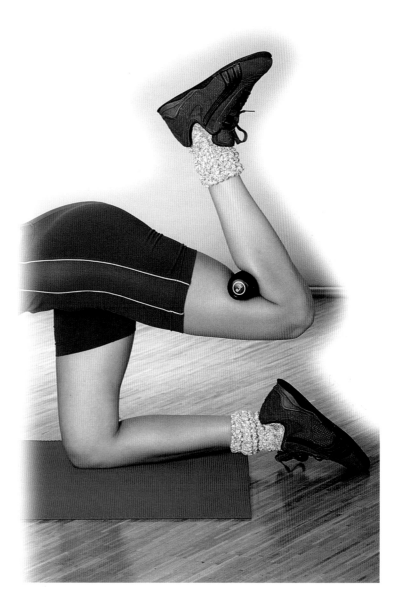

Leg Opener on Back

- For this exercise you will need resistance tubing.
- Start by lying down on your back. To avoid too much pressure on your lumbar spine, you should place your hands under your buttocks for support.
- Lift your legs up. Pull your toes toward your kneecap; knees remain slightly bent.
- To increase your physical stability, slightly tighten your abs.
- Slowly open your legs wide apart and close them again. This exercise is most effective if you do not close your legs completely but, instead, keep your feet apart about 1 foot (30 centimeters).

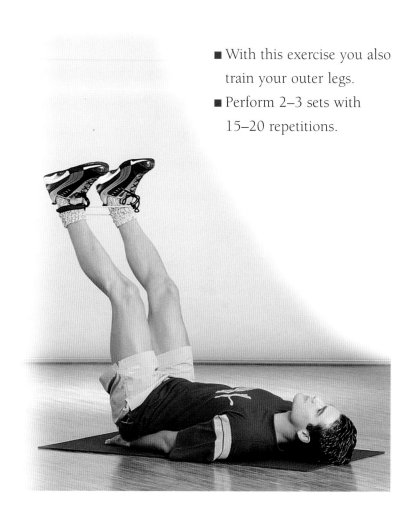

- With this exercise you also train your outer legs.
- Perform 2–3 sets with 15–20 repetitions.

Info

To avoid stiffness you should keep your head and shoulders on the floor at all times.

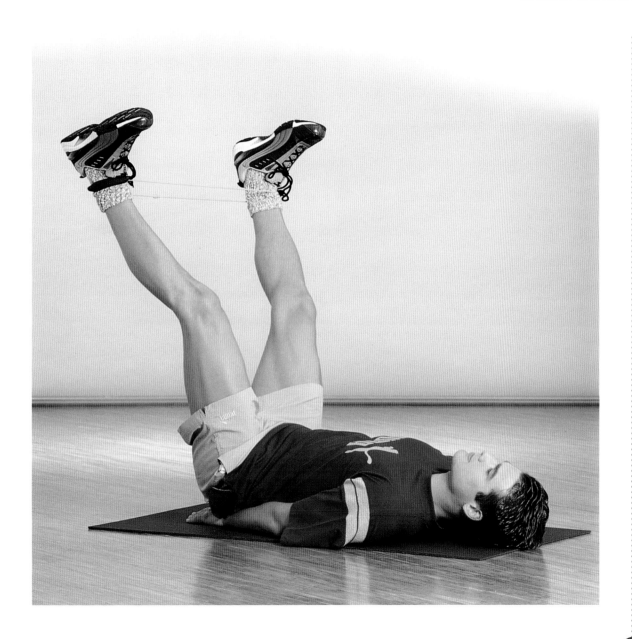

Shoulder Bridge

- Lie on your back, with your bent legs resting on your heels.
- Place your hands lightly on your stomach.
- Tighten your glutes and slowly lift up your pelvis while holding the tension in your buttocks.
- Move your pelvis back down and stop before you reach the floor.

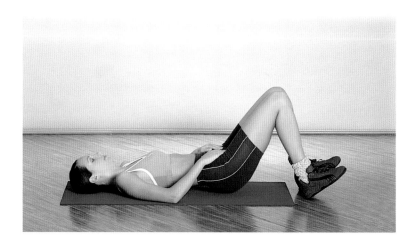

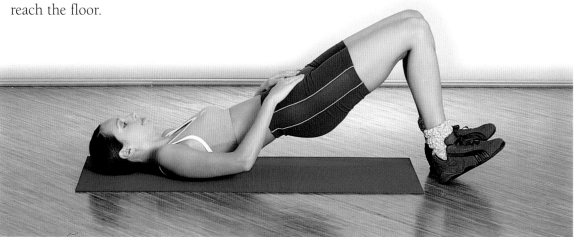

Variation

- If you place one or two hand weights on your groin, you will increase the level of difficulty.

- With this exercise you also train your posterior upper thigh muscles.
- Perform 2–3 sets with 15–20 repetitions.

Info

Make sure that your head, shoulders, and upper back remain firmly on the floor.

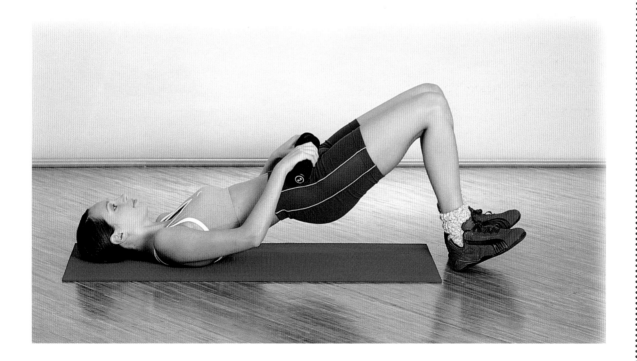

Lunges

- Stand upright and take a big lunge forward. Position the Thera-Band underneath your front leg. Take the loose ends into your hands. Stretch the band and make sure that it is tight at all times.
- Bend your front leg and inhale.
- Extend your leg again and exhale.

Tip

When you no longer have a problem with your balance after a few sessions, change the surface on which you exercise. For instance, place your front and rear leg on a pillow. This way you can further improve your body control.

- Afterward, switch your legs.
- With this exercise you can really tone your glutes while at the same time practicing your coordination and balance.

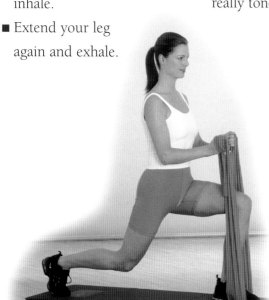

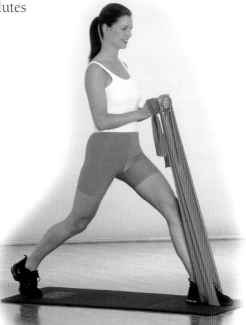

Lying Leg Press

- Lie on your back with your head resting on a flat pillow.
- Bend one leg and pull it toward your chest. The other leg remains extended on the floor during the entire exercise. Wrap the Thera-Band around your pulled-up leg and place the loose ends of the band next to your body.
- Extend your leg upward against the resistance of the band. Exhale deeply.
- During this exercise you will feel a tension in your leg muscles and glutes. At the same time, an intense stretch can be felt in the back of your upper thigh.
- Switch sides.

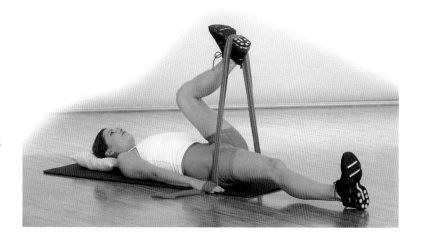

Info

During this exercise it is necessary that you always check your breathing.

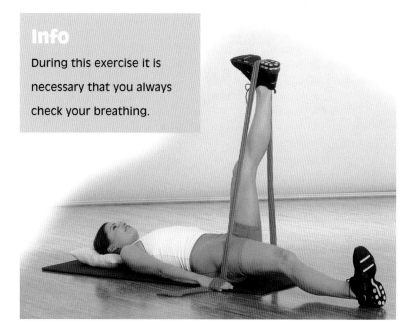

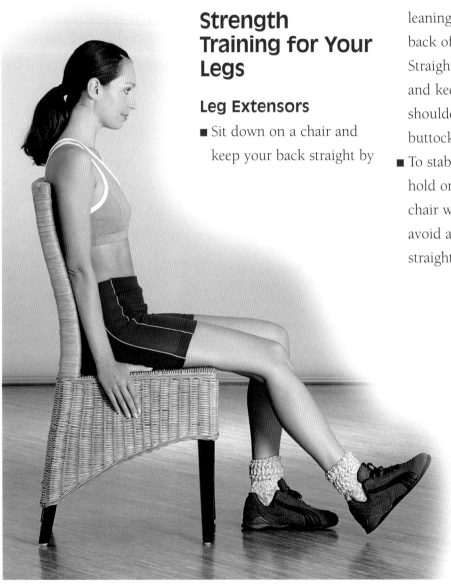

Strength Training for Your Legs

Leg Extensors

■ Sit down on a chair and keep your back straight by leaning firmly against the back of the chair. Straighten your chest bone and keep pulling your shoulders toward your buttocks.

■ To stabilize your torso, hold onto the sides of the chair with both hands. To avoid a stiff neck, look straight ahead.

■ Extend and bend one leg without placing your foot on the floor. The backs of your upper thighs should maintain contact with your seat. Your toes should be pulled toward your knees.

Variation

■ By using an exercise handle, you will increase the intensity of this exercise. Be aware that this variation requires a great deal of strength. Only perform this exercise if you feel completely familiar with its technical execution.

■ Do not forget to switch legs during the exercise.

■ Perform 2–3 sets with 15–20 repetitions, depending on your fitness level.

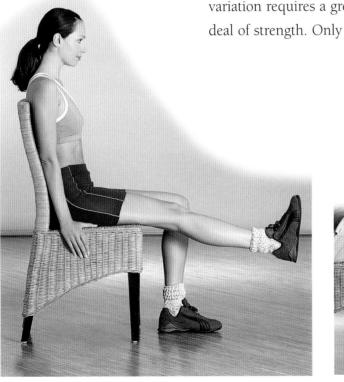

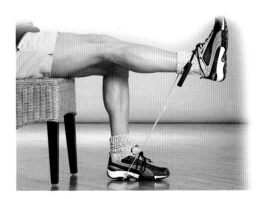

Exercises for Your Inner Thighs

Frog

- Start by lying on your back. To avoid too much strain on your lumbar spine, place your hands under your buttocks for support.
- Lift your legs up with your toes, knees pointing outward. Pull your toes toward your knees so that your soles face the ceiling.
- Pull your knee joints down toward your shoulder joints, knees slightly turned outward.
- Move back to the starting position. Your head remains on the floor at all times during the exercise.
- Perform 2–3 sets with 15–20 repetitions.

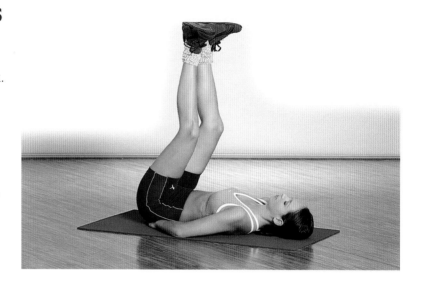

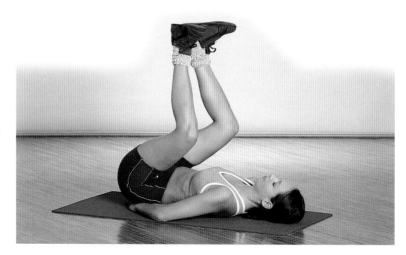

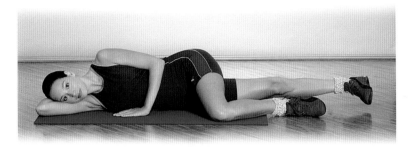

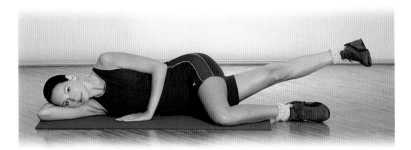

Strengthening Your Inner Thighs on Your Side

- Lie on your side, with your lower leg almost extended and your toes pointing forward.
- Your upper leg is bent and rests above the lower leg in front of your body. Turn your pelvis so that you do not lie on your hips.
- Lift your lower leg without momentum and slowly move it back to the starting position without allowing it to touch the floor.
- Switch legs.

Variation

- Use an exercise handle to increase resistance.
- Perform 2–3 sets with 15–20 repetitions per leg.

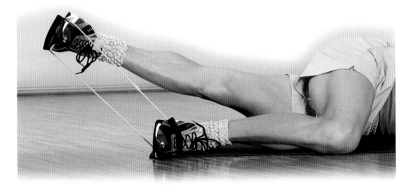

Strengthening Your Inner Thighs While Lying on Your Back

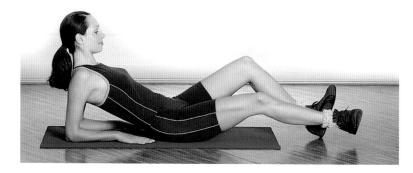

- Lie on your back and support your torso with your forearms.

- Slightly bend your left leg and place it on the floor. Your right knee and the toes of your right foot point outward.

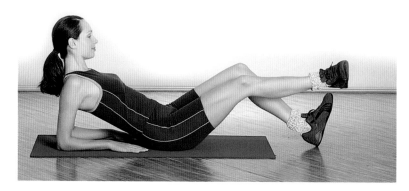

- Keep your back straight by pushing your chest bone forward and pulling your shoulder blades toward your buttocks. Your head remains still and your eyes look straight ahead.

- Lift and lower your right, slightly bent leg without letting it touch the floor. Make sure that your toes always point outward during this exercise.

- Do not forget to switch legs.

Variation

- Use an exercise handle to increase the intensity of the exercise.

- Perform 2–3 sets with 15–20 repetitions, depending on your fitness level.

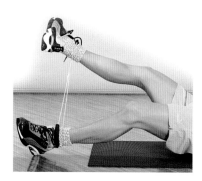

Wide Squat

- Open your legs wide with your knees and toes pointing outward.
- Support your torso with your hands resting on your upper thighs and keep your back straight and firm during this exercise.
- Push your buttocks down and back, as if sitting down in a chair. Do not push your knees forward. Your weight should rest solely on your heels during the entire exercise.
- Move back to the starting position.

- With this exercise you also shape your glutes. (For more squats, see pages 90 to 93.)
- Perform 2–3 sets with 15–20 repetitions, depending on your fitness level.

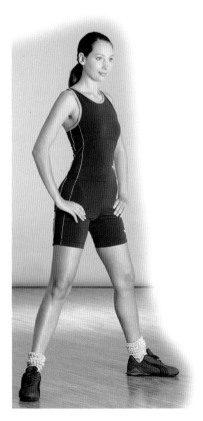

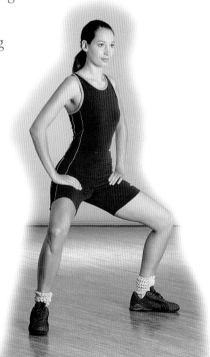

Exercises for Your Outer Thighs

Reverse Lunge

- Stand with legs shoulder-width apart.
- Take a big step back with your right leg without

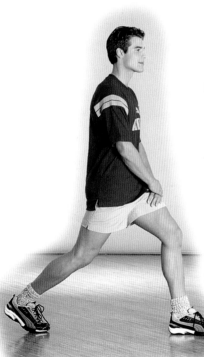

touching the floor with your right heel. Make sure to keep your torso upright. Your eyes should look straight ahead at all times.

- To support your torso, rest your hands on the upper thigh of your slightly bent front leg. Your chest bone remains straight and your shoulders are pulled toward your buttocks.
- Slightly bend your right knee, lower your body, and lift it up again. Your weight should be on the heels of your front leg. During this exercise, keep your back straight and firm.
- Remember to switch legs.

Info

In order to avoid knee problems, do not push the knee of your front leg forward. A 90-degree angle serves as an ideal starting position for the knee of your front leg.

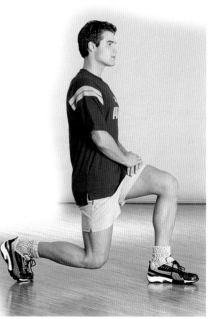

Variation

■ You can also perform this exercise by constantly alternating between left and right leg.

■ To intensify the exercise we recommend using hand weights on your shoulders.

■ This variation demands a great deal of physical stability (balance). You should only perform this exercise once you are completely familiar with the reverse lunge.

■ With this exercise you will also train your anterior and posterior upper thigh muscles.

■ Perform 2–3 sets with 15–20 repetitions per leg, depending on your fitness level.

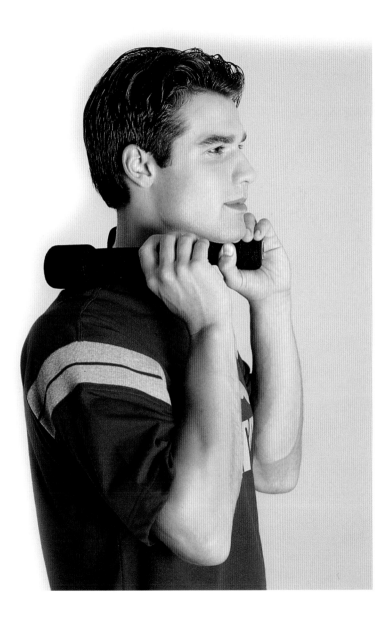

Exercises for Your Calf Muscles

Calf Raise

- Stand upright with your legs shoulder-width apart. Your toes and knees point forward. To keep your balance, use a chair for support.
- Shift your weight onto the balls of your feet and lift your heels off the floor.
- Slowly lower your heels again without letting them touch the floor. Your knees should remain slightly bent during the entire exercise.
- Depending on your fitness level, we recommend 2–3 sets with 15–20 repetitions.

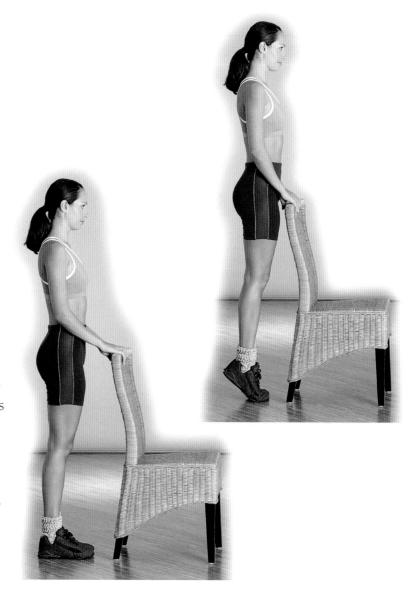

Downhill Position

- Stand with your legs hip-width apart and bend your legs until your buttocks and knees are on the same level.

- During this exercise make sure that your knees always remain behind the tips of your toes and that your weight rests on your heels.
- Start to rock slightly and shift your weight from the left to the right and then back to the starting position. Remember to switch sides.

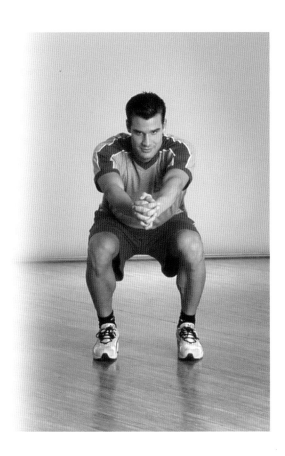

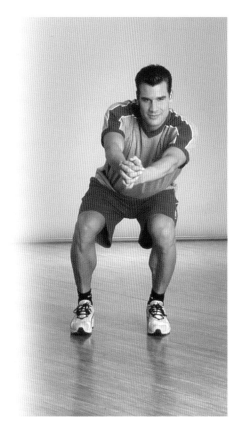

Thera-Band Workout

Quite a number of the strength training exercises on the previous pages can also be performed or intensified with a Thera-Band. Thera-Bands are perfect for your daily workout. Because they are small and light, they can be carried along anywhere. Whether in your office, at home, or on vacation— nothing should stand in the way of your workout!

Tip

In order to enjoy your band for a long time, keep in mind the following points: After your workout do not place your band on a heating device to let it dry. Rather, hang it over a chair and fold it. Do not leave your band tied up in knots. Clean it with water and sprinkle talcum powder on it after use. Check your band regularly for any small holes.

Choose your own level of difficulty. The color of the band indicates its level of resistance. Dark colors stand for a high level of resistance, whereas light colors indicate a lower level of resistance. Ideally, you should buy two bands with different resistances so that you can perform the exercises with varying levels of difficulty. A Thera-Band with a length of at least 5 feet (150 centimeters) has proven to be the most effective. You may vary the length of the band by tying knots or placing a clip in it.

Squat

- Stand upright with your legs hip width apart. Turn the tips of your toes lightly outward and place the band with its loose ends under your feet.

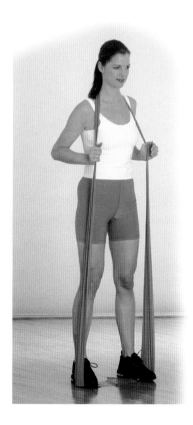

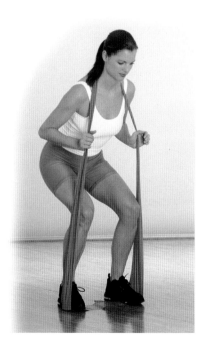

- Slip your torso through the band so that it rests on your neck. Make sure the Thera-Band does not rest too high as it will put pressure on your cervical spine. Secure the band with your hands.
- Bend your hips and knees and inhale deeply during the movement.
- Extend both legs again and exhale deeply. Make sure you move with your knees, hips, and lower back.
- This exercise works your glutes and leg muscles.

Info

There is a close interrelationship between breathing and relaxation. Breathe slowly and evenly while you hold the stretch. Deep and complete breathing is a necessity for both physical fitness and inner harmony.

Stretching

The final part of your workout session serves to stretch and relax your muscles as well as to provide both physical and mental relaxation. Play calm, relaxing music and make sure to keep the volume at a comfortable level. Stretching effectively prevents your muscles from becoming stiff and tense.

Please Be Aware!

- All working muscles have to be stretched.
- Hold each stretch for about 20–30 seconds.
- To achieve a successful result, do not rock during stretching.
- Do not overstretch your muscles. Often, less is more. During stretching you should feel a slight pull but no pain. Avoid extreme stretching to prevent injuries.

On Motivation

- Stretching is the last part of your workout session. Try to look forward to it in order to keep yourself motivated during your workout and to ensure that you start your next workout in a cheerful frame of mind.

The Advantages of Stretching

- Stretching increases your range of motion. With the help of a heightened sense of mobility, you will perform everyday activities faster, more easily, and more economically.
- By gaining control of the body through regular stretching you will learn new movements more easily.

Correct Stretching

- Start to stretch slowly to make sure that your muscles and the linear measuring instruments of your muscles (neuromuscular spindles) can adapt to the extension. End your stretching just as slowly as you started it.

- After about 6–8 seconds, there are fewer signals of the neuromuscular spindles firing. You will feel this in the form of decreased muscle tension. You may then intensify the stretch a bit and hold the position for another 10–20 seconds. Even at this point, start with caution and intensify your stretching slowly to avoid a pulled muscle.

- Exhale while you start to stretch.

- Try to feel the contraction and relaxation of your muscles.

- Stretches should be repeated 2–3 times.

- Make sure that the room in which you stretch is warm enough while also providing fresh air. In open air you should limit your stretching to standing exercises.

- Keep in mind correct posture while you stretch.

- Make sure to stretch both sides of your body.

Stretching Helps

- Release tension within your body, which improves your overall well-being
- Achieve physical relaxation and inner harmony
- Increase physical and mental fitness
- Reduce the risk of injury
- Normalize your muscle tone after working out
- Avoid strained muscles and soreness

Tip

The following stretches can be performed without a prior workout. Take some time every day and put together your favorite exercises. Regardless of when you stretch, warm up 5 minutes at the beginning.

For Biceps and Pectorals

- Stand next to a door frame or a wall. Rest your palm on the wall at right angles to your torso.

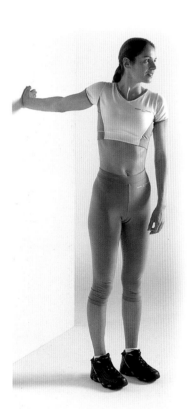

- Slowly turn your body away from your extended arm.
- Switch sides. Turning away your head will intensify the stretch.

For Arm and Biceps

- You may perform this stretch standing or sitting.
- Keep your torso upright and straight.
- Extend your right arm forward and pull down your shoulders. Only in this particular position will you have to stretch your elbows completely.
- Place your left hand on the ball of your right hand and push the hand down. Your wrist forms a straight line with your arm and should not be overstretched.

- Hold the stretch while breathing calmly and evenly.
- Do not forget to switch arms.

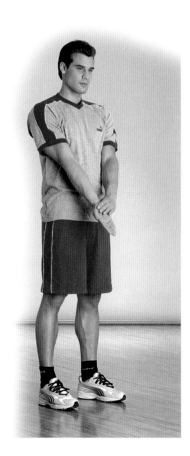

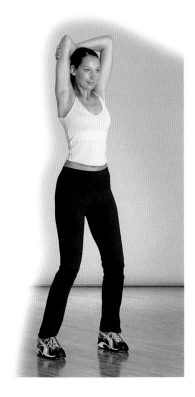

For Arm and Triceps

- Stand or sit with your torso upright.
- Bend your right arm and move it behind your head so that your hand is positioned between your shoulder blades.

- With your left hand, grab the back side of your upper arm and gently push it behind your head. Straighten your head and look straight ahead. Try to relax your neck. Also make sure to keep your back straight and avoid a hollow back.
- Hold this stretch 20–30 seconds and then switch arms.

For Your Shoulder

- Stand upright with your knees slightly bent. Extend your right arm to the left

and pull it close to your body with your left hand while your shoulder is pulled down.
- Do not forget to switch arms.

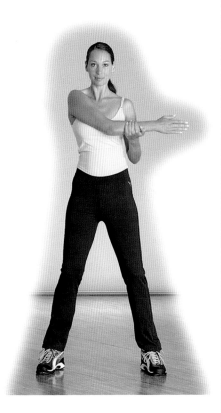

For Chest and Shoulder

- Stand upright with your knees slightly bent. Your neck and shoulders are relaxed.

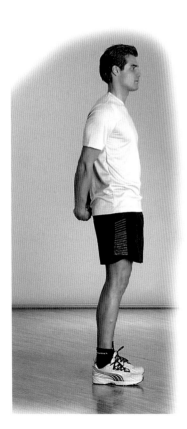

- Cross your hands behind your back but keep your elbows slightly bent.
- Pull down your arms and shoulders, with your head and back forming a straight line, and straighten your chest bone.

For Your Chest

- Start from the same position as in the stretch for chest and shoulders. In contrast to the chest and shoulder stretch, slightly bend the arms that are crossed behind your back and lift them up a bit.
- Remember to breathe calmly and evenly.

Info

With this exercise you also stretch the front part of your shoulder muscles.

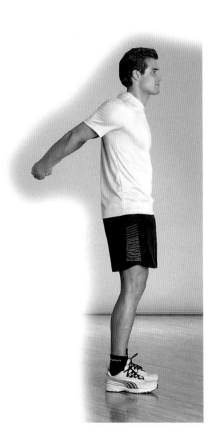

For Your Neck

■ Sit up straight and push down your right shoulder.

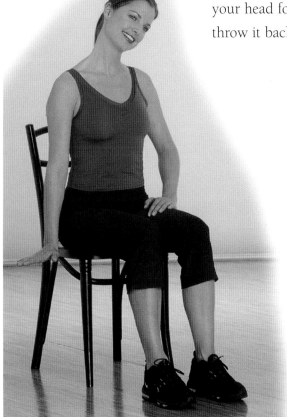

Lean your head to the left until you feel the stretch on the right side of your neck.

■ Your eyes should look straight ahead. Do not bow your head forward or throw it back.

Info

You can easily perform stretches during breaks at work! Try to stretch your tense muscles several times a day.

■ Pay attention to your breathing. Exhaling has an intensifying effect on your stretch.

■ Hold the position for 30 seconds and then switch sides.

■ You can also perform this exercise standing.

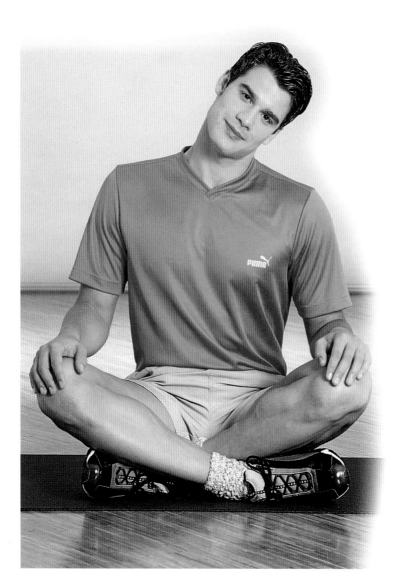

Sitting Variation

- The stretches for neck and throat are good balance exercises for anyone sitting at a desk for long hours.
- Sit down on your exercise mat with your back straight and your shoulders pulled down and relaxed. Place your hands on your knees.
- Move your head to the left. Make sure that your torso remains straight during the entire exercise.

Variation A

- Perform this exercise the same as you have the neck stretch on the previous page, but do not move your head to the left; look down to your left knee.

Tip

Do not forget to switch sides during the stretch and variation A.

Variation B

- The starting position is the same as in the neck stretch.
- Pull your chin toward your chest to stretch the posterior neck muscles.

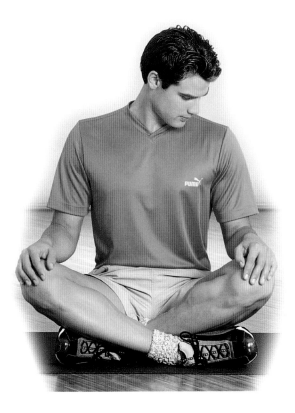

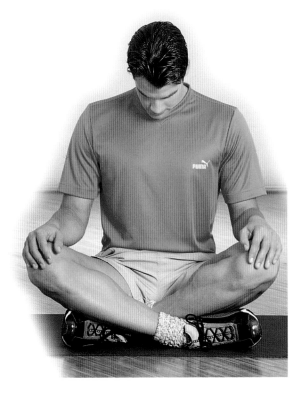

For Upper and Lower Back Muscles

- Go down on all fours and balance your weight equally on knees and hands. To avoid unnecessary pressure on your elbows and shoulders, leave your elbows slightly bent. Your back remains straight.
- Push up your back as if it were being pulled up by a string, and arch your back. Pull in your stomach. Do not forget to breathe evenly during the stretch.
- Slowly move your stomach back toward the floor.

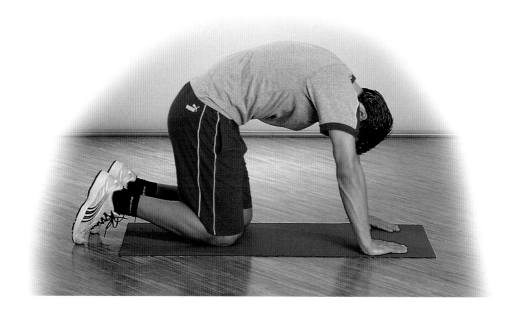

For Your Upper Back Muscles

- Sit down on a chair and imagine you are hugging a big tree in front of you.
- Cross your hands, with your palms facing your body.
- Your shoulders are pulled down and your elbows are slightly bent.
- Open your shoulder blades and slightly pull in your chest. Bow your head toward your chest a bit.

Variation

- You can also cross your arms in front of you and grab your shoulders in the back. Round your upper back and pull your shoulders forward. Your head is again slightly bowed down.

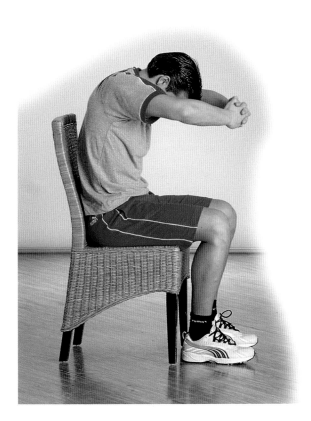

Info

Remember to breathe calmly and evenly.

For Your Back Muscles

- Sit down with your legs slightly bent and open; push your torso forward.

- Wrap your arms around your legs from the inside out.

- Roll in your torso and move your chin toward your chest. You can move your legs slightly forward to intensify the stretch. Remember to breathe evenly.

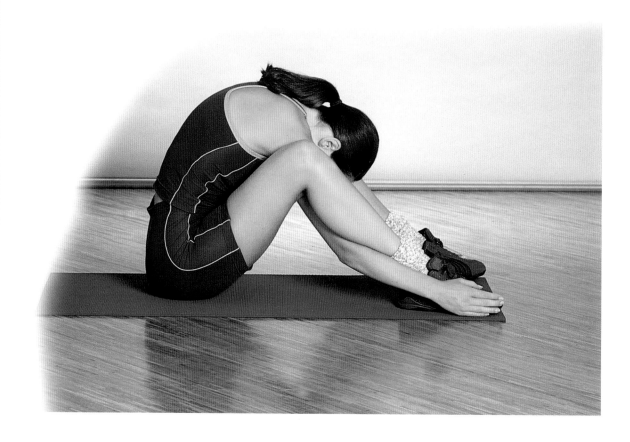

For Your Oblique Abdominal Muscles

- Lie on your back and place both feet on the floor. Extend your arms like the wings of an airplane next to your body. Your palms face the ceiling.

- Move both bent legs to the left and turn your head to the right. Both shoulder blades remain on the floor. Inhale and exhale consciously during the stretch.

- During this exercise do not forget to switch sides.

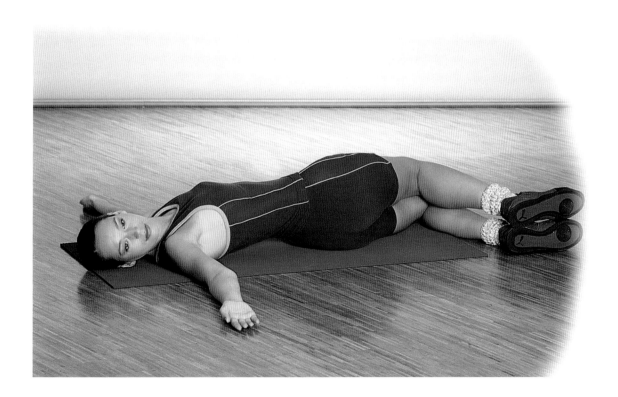

For Your Abdominal muscles

- Lie flat on your back. Stretch your legs out and extend your arms above your head.
- Close your eyes, breathe calmly, and concentrate your thoughts on your stretching.
- During the stretch imagine someone holding you by your hands and feet and slowly pulling you apart.

Info

Lying on the floor provides an optimal position for relaxation, since our body does not put anything in the way of gravity.

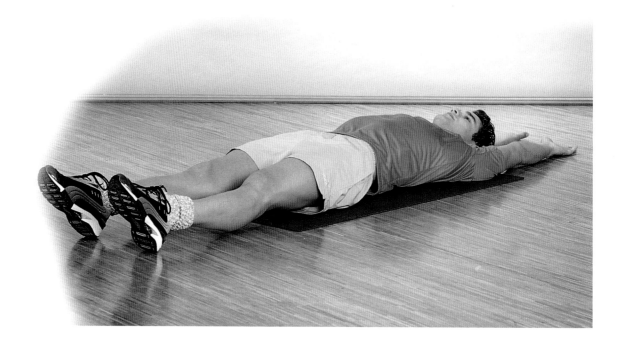

Stretch 1 for Your Glutes

- Lie on your back and rest both feet on the floor.
- Wrap your arms around your shins and pull your knees to your body. Your head, shoulders, and upper back remain on the floor during the entire exercise.

Info

During this exercise you will also stretch your lower back.

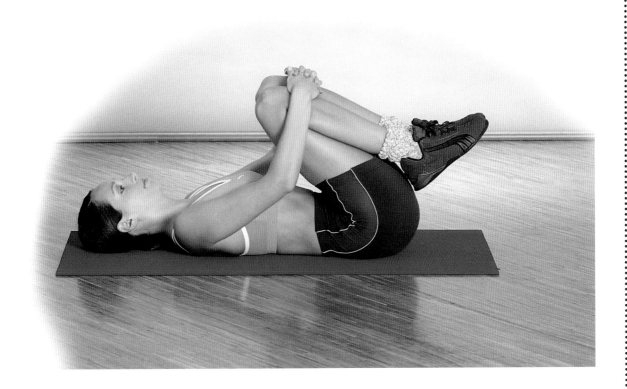

Stretch 2 for Your Glutes

- Use the same starting position as in stretch 1 on page 131.
- Lay your right foot on your left upper thigh and turn the right knee slightly outward.
- Wrap both arms around the back of your left upper thigh and pull your leg toward your body. Your head, shoulders, and upper back remain on the floor during the whole stretch.
- Do not forget to switch legs.

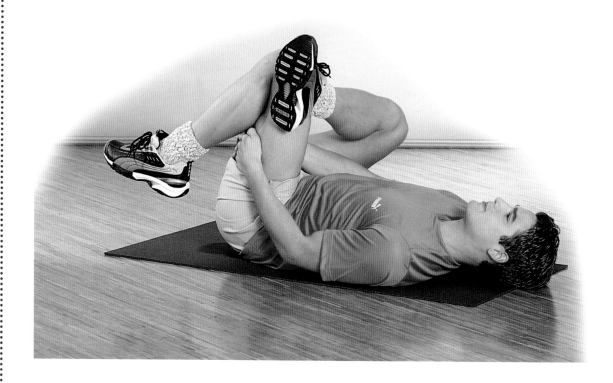

For Your Calves

- Standing upright, move one leg far behind you. Both heels touch the floor and your feet are parallel to each other.

- Your arms rest on the upper thigh of your front leg. During this exercise make sure to keep your back firm and straight. Your body should form a straight line from your head to your rear heel. Make sure that your front knee is not pushed beyond the tips of your toes and that the knee of your rear leg is slightly bent.

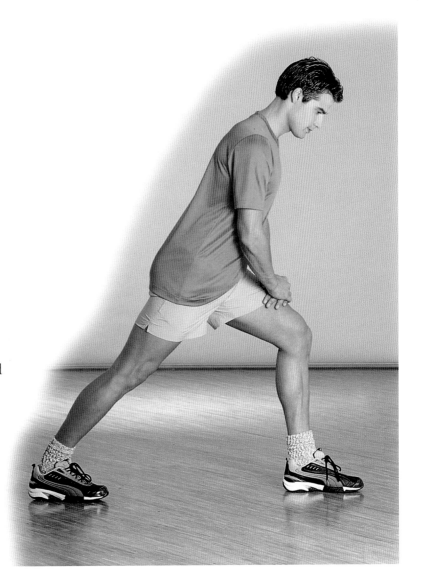

For Your Anterior Leg Muscles

- To keep your balance, hold onto a chair during this stretch. Stand on your left leg, with your knee slightly bent.
- Grab your right heel with your right hand and push your bent leg back while pushing your hip forward. Your heel does not touch your buttocks. Make sure to keep your upper thighs parallel to each other.

Info

If you want, you can perform this exercise lying on your side.

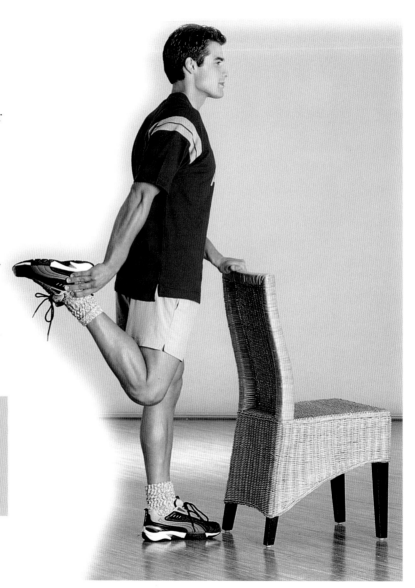

Variation

■ Start with a lunge and rest your rear leg on your knee.

■ Grab the back of your foot and pull your heel toward your buttocks. You will feel a stretch on the front of your upper thigh.

■ Hold this position for about 30 seconds and then switch sides.

Tips

■ Perform the stretch on a mat or place a pillow under your knee.

■ If necessary hold on to a chair.

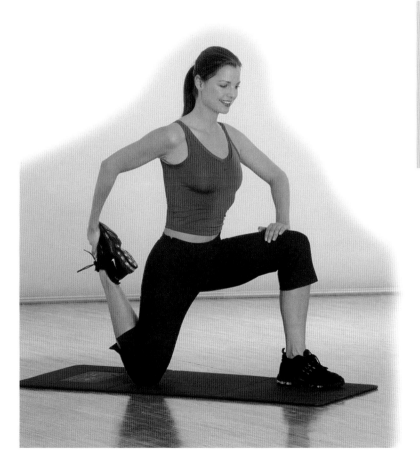

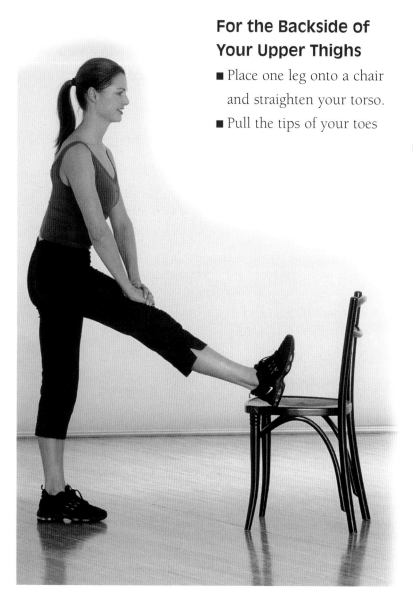

For the Backside of Your Upper Thighs

- Place one leg onto a chair and straighten your torso.
- Pull the tips of your toes toward your shin and slightly bow down your torso. You will feel a distinct stretch on the back of your upper thighs.
- Hold the stretch for about 30 seconds and then switch legs.

For Your Posterior Leg Muscles

- Lying on your back, place both feet on the floor.
- Lift up your left leg.
- Wrap both hands around your left leg, which is extended toward the ceiling, and slowly pull your leg toward your body. Your head and shoulders remain on the floor at all times.

- Perform this stretch gently and carefully, as injuries are possible.

Tip

You can also use a towel as an extension of your arms.

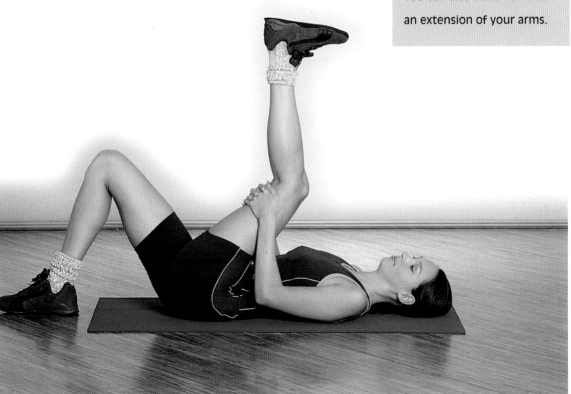

For Your Outer Thighs

- Lie on your back and extend your arms like the wings of an airplane next to your body. Your palms should face the ceiling.
- Bend your left knee and place it sideways over your extended right leg.
- Your right hand rests on the upper thigh of your left leg. During this stretch your head and back always remain on the floor.

Info

People suffering from damaged discs should not perform this stretch.

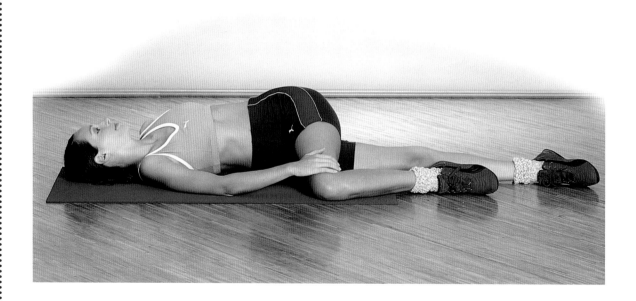

For Your Inner Thighs

- Lie on your back. Pull both knees toward your chest and then open your legs.

- Extend your legs outward and pull your toes toward your knees to intensify the stretch.

- Your hands rest on the inside of your upper thighs. Your head, shoulders, and back always remain on the floor.

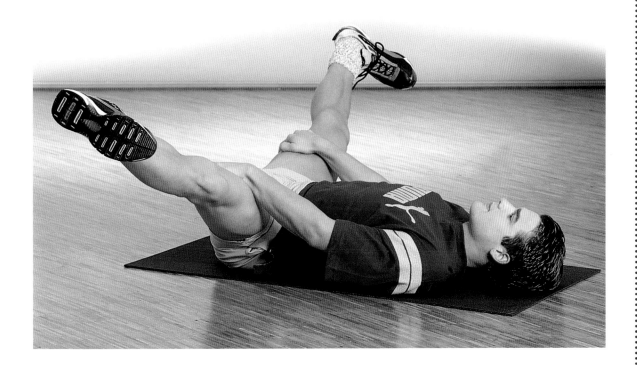

Side Stretches

- Extend your right arm high above your head and slightly bend your torso to the left.
- Hold this position for about 30 seconds and then switch sides.
- Try to extend your arm a bit more each time you inhale.
- Perform this stretch several times on each side.

Info

With these body stretching exercises, you simultaneously activate your abs and back muscles.

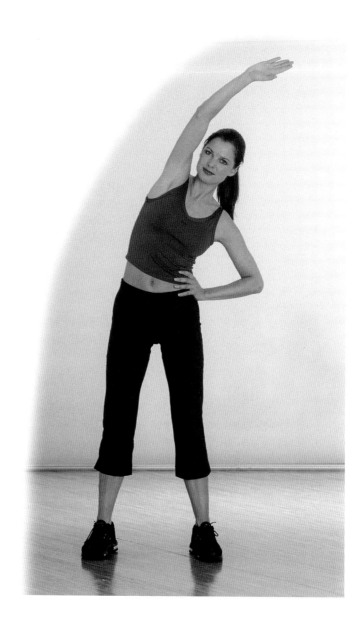

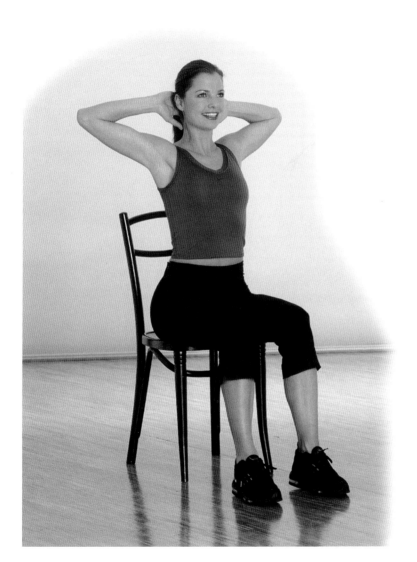

For your torso

■ Cross your hands behind your head and forcefully push your elbows back. Hold the stretch for about 10 seconds.

■ Release the tension, relax for 20–30 seconds, and then repeat the exercise several times.

Info

For big-chested women, stretching the pectorals and strengthening the back muscles is particularly important.

Cool-down

Dedicate the last phase of your workout to relaxing. Just concentrate on yourself!

- Lie on a comfortable surface and use a blanket to cover yourself, if you like. Rest your head and knees on a pillow or a rolled up towel.
- Extend your arms slightly away from your body with your palms facing up. Close your eyes, if you like.
- Concentrate solely on your breathing. Specifically try to feel the exhalation. Feel how you relax with each breath.
- Remain in this position for a few minutes and continue to breathe evenly.
- Inhale deeply a few times, open your eyes, and slowly stand up.

Info

Do not get nervous if you have some trouble with the cool-down. With time and practice you will really enjoy it!

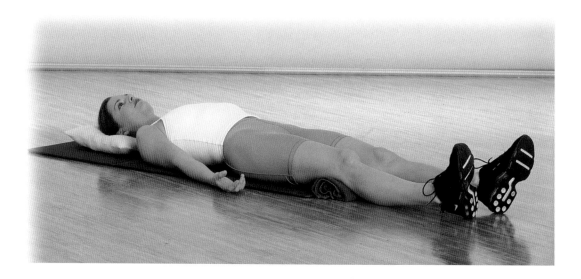

4 Endurance Workout

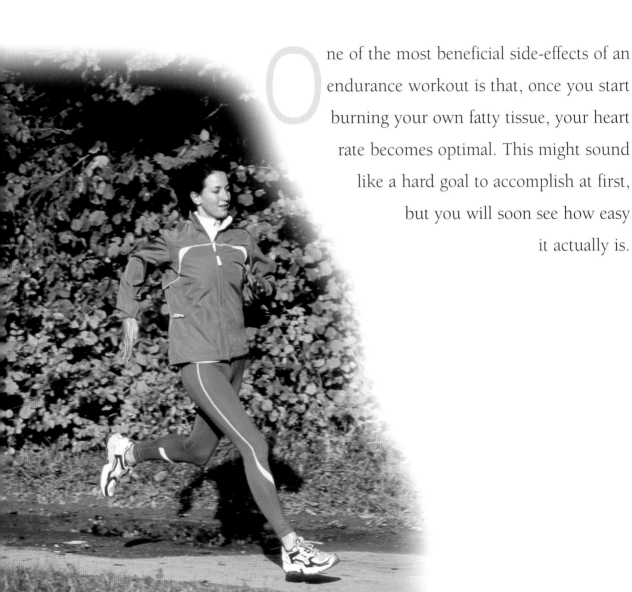

One of the most beneficial side-effects of an endurance workout is that, once you start burning your own fatty tissue, your heart rate becomes optimal. This might sound like a hard goal to accomplish at first, but you will soon see how easy it actually is.

Fat-burning Endurance Workout

A fat-burning endurance workout is often called a cardiovascular workout. Endurance should not be confused with physical fitness, as physical fitness entails not only endurance but also strength, flexibility, speed, and coordination. Endurance indicates how long someone can perform a physical exercise without tiring. There is a difference between aerobic and anaerobic endurance workouts. An aerobic endurance workout provides the body with enough oxygen to burn sources of energy. The level of intensity chosen for this type of workout allows for enough oxygen to be transported to the muscles and then used as a source of energy. Where there is increased stress, oxygen alone is not sufficient to provide the necessary energy. For this

- Enjoy your workout. Choose your favorite type of endurance sport or some workout gear that you especially like.
- If you start your workout past the age of 35, you should first see a doctor for a physical checkup.
- Do not engage in any endurance sport if you have an infectious disease. Once you have recovered, continue your workout slowly, step by step.
- Use a device to measure your heart rate.
- Work out regularly. Try to perform your workout sessions several times a week, in keeping with your schedule.
- Increase the time and intensity of your workout slowly, according to your own personal preference.

reason the body will create energy by producing lactic acid (lactate).

Apart from toned muscles, body weight is an important aspect of body styling. Perhaps you have had the experience of losing weight through diets and then regaining it even faster as soon as the diet was over. This yo-yo effect takes place because our bodies start to save energy during calorie reduction, thus slowing down our metabolism. Once you start to eat regularly again, you will find not everything can be burned on account of a slower metabolism and because the body has been storing fat. A harsh truth is that weight loss during diets is often

caused by a loss of muscle mass. By contrast, an endurance workout has a different effect, and with correct nutrition becomes a real "fat burner." Through regular cardio workout the body starts to systematically burn fat. This does not happen at once, because the body first needs to adjust to the endurance workout. However, after 4–8 weeks of such a program fat is burned at full speed.

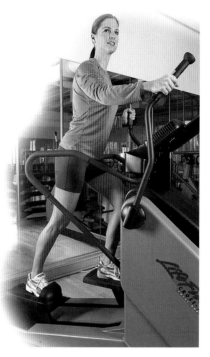

Indoors or Outdoors

Whether you perform your endurance training outside in fresh air or at home with the help of an endurance training device—a treadmill or an ergometer, for instance—is up to you. What

is important is that you choose the right intensity and duration of your workout. Of course you may also choose an indoor sport during the cold season and train outdoors during the warmer months.

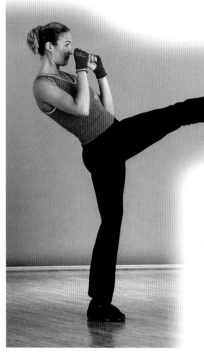

Aerobics

Today, aerobics has become a generic term for numerous gym classes that are offered in fitness studios. Yet, only courses that offer real endurance exercise are suited for burning fat. They may be called step aerobics, low impact, fat burner, calorie burner, or thai-bo. These courses aim mainly at improving flexibility and, of course, at effectively burning fat. Motivational music, group motivation, and a qualified aerobics instructor will transform each workout into a great experience. To ensure long-lasting joy with this sport consider the following tips:

■ For aerobic workouts that protect your joints, well-cushioned sneakers are necessary to provide your feet with stability and shock absorption. Definitely get some advice from a qualified sports outfitter. Wearing new shoes a couple of hours each day before your first workout session will avoid painful blisters.

■ Comfortable clothing is a key. Whether you follow fashion trends or whether you prefer a classic outfit is up to your personal taste. Clothing made of fibers that do not close off body heat but transport it away from the body ensures that your body will not get overheated.

■ Beginners should choose classes that do not include jumps, since they put too much pressure on the joints and on the cardiovascular system. Using technical terms, this is called "low impact."

Walking

Fast walking has developed into a very popular sport in the United States. Walking hardly affects any joints and is a gentle workout for the buttocks and legs. The impact load on the musculoskeletal system is much lower than with jogging. For this reason walking is especially suitable for overweight people and beginners. Through this gentle movement of the entire body, your metabolism is stimulated to burn fat. The

correct heart rate is important. For your warm-up, start walking slowly and rotate your shoulders every so often. Keep your back straight and look straight ahead. After about 5 minutes, increase your speed and your arm movements. Consciously roll your feet forcefully from

heel to toe. Hand weights held tightly in your hands may increase the intensity of your workout.

Jogging

The advantages of jogging are that it is easy to learn, it can be done pretty much

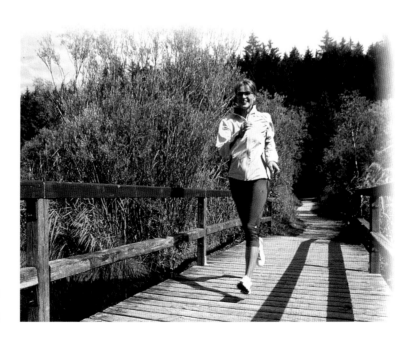

anywhere and at anytime, and it is relatively easy and cheap—all you need is a good pair of running shoes.

Tips for Buying Shoes

- Beginners should value solid footwear to prevent problems during running and to reduce the impact load.
- A detailed consultation at a specialized store is a must! A competent salesperson will pay attention to the formation of your foot and your

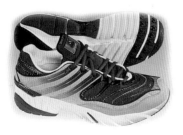

weight in order to find a shoe with an appropriate insole.

- Take your old shoes to the store with you. Sole abrasion shows your individual running style or a possible indisposition of the foot.
- A good running shoe should fit like a glove, even when you first try it on. It should not pinch or squeeze your foot.

Clothing

If you run regularly, weatherproof fitness clothing will pay off. As we mentioned before, you always want to avoid a heat buildup. For this reason wear fibers that transmit heat out of your body.

Cycling

Since your body weight rests on the seat of a bicycle, cycling is a very good sport for beginners, people who are overweight, or for those with joint problems. Due to

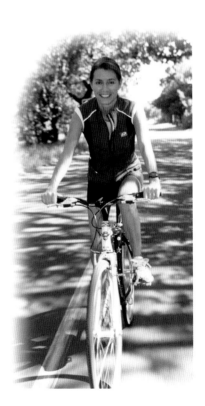

its simple movement and load control, cycling is suitable also for those who have been inactive for a while. Clothing that fits tightly and covers the lower back protects from hypothermia. Wear an additional breathable jacket if necessary. Specially padded cycling pants are certainly not necessary for your first few trips, but as soon as you start to train regularly this very useful piece of clothing will pay off. Cycling pants prevent beginners and pros alike from chafing the upper thighs, feeling pain on your pelvis, and experiencing genital numbness.

Swimming

Swimming is an endurance sport that is also recommended for overweight people. The buoyancy of the water leads to significant weight reduction. The pressure on the joints is reduced to a minimum due to a lack of impact load. Since the body

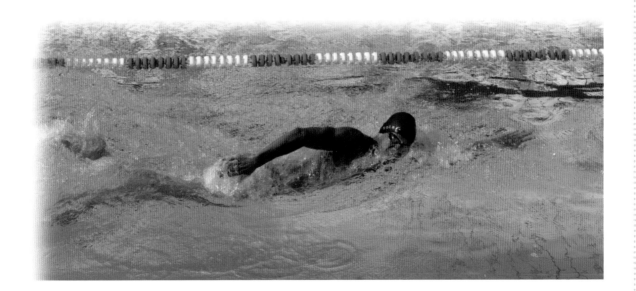

receives permanent cooling through the water, sweating is limited. There is not much to say about equipment—most people own a swimsuit and a towel. If swimming develops into a passion, then goggles are recommended to protect the eyes from chemicals in indoor and outdoor swimming pools. Some indoor pools also offer

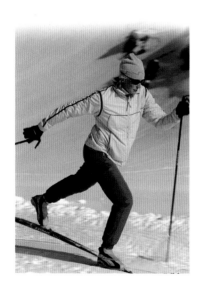

a number of devices for rent, such as boogie boards, fins, and paddles, which can be included in your swim training to ensure variety or to practice specific movements.

Cross-country Skiing

Due to its sliding movements, cross-country skiing is a sport that protects your joints. Movements performed by the whole body have an impact on numerous muscles. For beginners, we recommend buying used skiing equipment, but if you plan to immerse yourself in cross-country skiing, it is advisable to find a

specialized dealer where you can get detailed information and advice on suitable equipment. It is also recommended that you take a beginner level course at a local ski school where you will learn the correct techniques and receive useful advice for a workout that will be a lot of fun!

SPORT	USE IN KCAL/ HOUR
Aerobics	approx. 550
Step-aerobics	approx. 500
Hiking	approx. 750
Jogging	approx. 650
Cycling	approx. 600
Rowing	approx. 750
Swimming	approx. 450
Cross-country skiing	approx. 750

Heart Rate

Once you know which intensity and duration of a workout helps you to best burn fat, you can systematically start to lose weight. Do not forget, however, that your body needs sufficient liquids to keep functioning.

Heart Rate—Less Is More

Beginners often have a hard time finding the right workout intensity. Due to physical exhaustion, beginners often lose their initial motivation and end up dropping the workout during the first few days. In this context a training heart rate that is too high will

actually do more harm than good. If you want to lose weight, the workout intensity, measured with the help of the training heart rate, will be significant for your success.

How High Can the Training Heart Rate Be?

As the old saying goes, many roads lead to Rome. There are just as many formulas to calculate the ideal training heart rate. In the end, all lead to the same result. The following formula provides a fast and easy way to calculate the average of one's individual training heart rate:

$$160 - age = $$
$$\text{average training heart rate}$$

Taking the example of a 35-year-old person, the following calculation is made:

$$160 - 35 = \text{average}$$
$$\text{training heart rate of 125}$$

Don't be fooled with this relatively low training heart rate and think that your workout is not strenuous enough. It is exactly the right intensity to provide for the sufficient flow of oxygen through correct and deep breathing, which is vital for burning fat. Moreover, through this relatively low training heart rate the blood also flows slowly enough to be able to provide all the important organs with nutrients via the capillary vessels and the inhaled fresh oxygen.

151

The Duration of Your Workout

During endurance workout, we achieve a maximum level of fat burning after about 30 minutes. For this reason, sessions of 30–60 minutes of health-oriented and fat-burning endurance workout present an ideal exercise period.

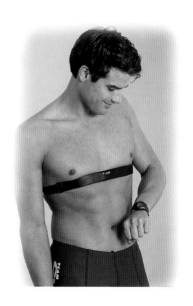

How to Control the Training Heart Rate

Since the training heart rate should be measured during physical exercise, it is recommended that you wear a heart rate monitor. The monitor consists of a transmitter and a receiver which allows you to monitor your heart rate constantly and safely via your running speed. Heart rate monitors are available in various models and features. Ask for more information at a specialized sports dealer.

How to Reach Your Training Heart Rate—the Warm-up

Scientific studies show that a warm-up physiologically leads to less impact on the body. The warm-up should vary depending on the main impact of the respective sport. For common endurance sports, such as jogging, cycling, swimming, or aerobics, a slow start is necessary. For cycling, this might mean relaxed cycling for 5–10 minutes. The intensity should be increased slowly with all endurance sports until the recommended training heart rate, also called the target zone, is reached. If the intensity is increased too fast or the training heart rate is reached too quickly, lactate levels will be too high, as the body is not ready yet. The consequences are painful muscle strains and a significantly longer rest period, which keeps you from further workout sessions.

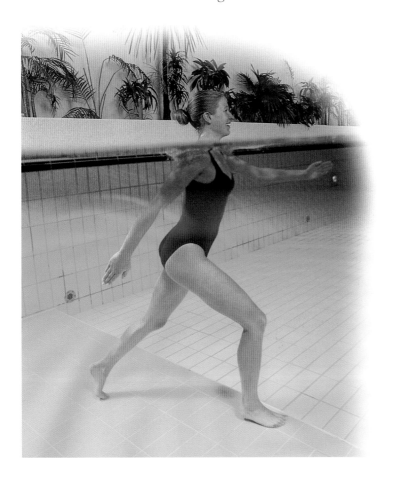

Monitoring the Impact

Planning an endurance workout depends on the goals of the exerciser. Our goal is to burn off excess fat.

Because of this the target zone, the main part of the workout should be maintained for at least 30 minutes. Which sport you wish to engage in to reach this goal is up to you. You definitely do not have to stick to only one sport. It is certainly possible to switch individual endurance sports daily or at specific intervals. Monitoring your own training heart rate, as we described on the previous page, is a very simple procedure. When cycling, you can increase your heart rate by riding up a hilly area or use hand weights when jogging. The sense of comfort you have during and after your workout will oftentimes determine

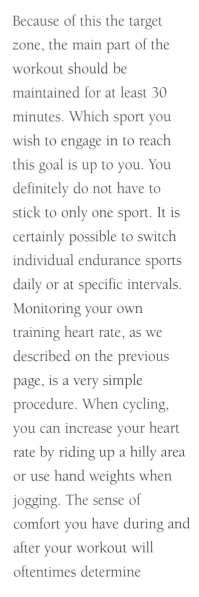

whether or not you will work out regularly. If you are completely exhausted, your workout was too intense. For almost all endurance sports you should train without breathing too hard. Choose a workout intensity that provides you with untroubled breathing and pay attention to how you feel. Remember, if you practice sports you will remain active for a long time.

From the Training Heart Rate to the Resting Heart Rate — the Cool-down

The cool-down is the third phase of a workout session and is the counterpart to the warm-up. It is very important and is divided into two phases.

When jogging, for example,

Phase 1 consists of slow running for about five minutes. This will break down the end products derived from your metabolism during the workout so that they can be excreted faster. Phase 1 also slowly reduces your body temperature and heart rate and marks the first step toward rest.

Phase 2 consists of stretching the main muscle

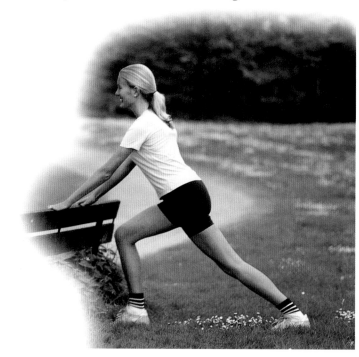

groups that were affected during the workout. This allows your muscles to maintain their flexibility and also restores your muscle tone to its original state. After the cool-down your heart rate should be as it was before exercising.

The Workout

To achieve a good ratio between body fat and lean body mass there has to be a good ratio between your eating habits and your workout program. The 7-calorie-rule serves here as a goal for additional use of energy. You use up 7 calories per 2 pounds (1 kilogram) of weight through an active lifestyle! An endurance workout is especially suitable for this, but also daily physical activity contributes significantly to a higher metabolism and increased use of calories. For instance, if you casually ride your bike for 10 minutes you use up 1 calorie per 2 pounds (1 kilogram) of weight. Please do not take on too much at once. Take small steps!

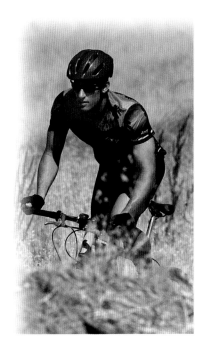

- On Mondays and Tuesdays I will not ride the escalator and I will not use the elevator anymore (during the course of 2–3 weeks add one additional day).
- For small errands such as going shopping I will walk or ride my bike.
- On the weekend I will not use the remote control anymore to switch TV channels.

Avoid dropout errors! In the following paragraphs you will find some ideas concerning planning and changing your daily life. Think of further opportunities to plan your life more actively step by step.

Planning Your Workout

Based on actively planning your daily life, the biggest success can be achieved through a systematic endurance workout and a change of diet. With sports that are fun you will hold out longer. For longer exercise periods, a combination of different aerobic workouts has proven very motivational. For instance, if you regularly visit a fitness studio or gym, you may design your workout as an endurance circuit with 5–15 minutes of cycling, step workout, and rowing. Outdoors you can ride your bike to the nearest lake or pool and then swim long enough to reach a workout duration. For fat-burning workouts there is a distinction between a minimum and an ideal workout.

Minimum Workout

A minimum workout describes the minimum amount of work that has to be performed to gain any significant positive effects. For the fat-burning workout, the minimum workout is characterized by the following features:

- Dynamic and endurance impact involving big muscle groups at a training heart rate of 160 minus your age.
- Duration of workout per week of about 60 minutes, divided among 2–3 days with 1–2 days of rest in between.

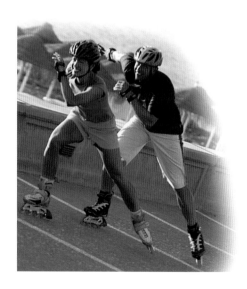

For beginners, the increase of physical fitness is very high at first. After several weeks you reach a plateau that can only be surpassed by increasing the duration of exercise.

The Ideal Workout

The ideal workout can only be determined on an individual basis. Once the increased level of exercise becomes disproportionate to any possible health improvement, we must rethink our workout regimen. For this ideal workout plan the criteria listed below are to be considered:

- Consistent and dynamic endurance workout involving major muscle groups at a training heart rate of 160 minus your age.
- Total workout duration per week of about 3–4 hours, divided among 4–5 workout days with 30–60 minutes per workout session.
- An extensive workout will improve physical fitness but will also ratchet up the effect at the same time. From a health point of view, this is neither necessary nor recommended for casual exercisers.

Tips for a Fat-burning Endurance Workout

- Exercise regularly! Only consistency leads to success! Long breaks between workouts quickly lead to a decrease in physical fitness.
- Exercise in a way that is enjoyable to you at all times.
- Do not exercise with a full stomach. The last big meal should be eaten at least 2 hours prior to your workout.
- Do not exercise on a completely empty stomach.

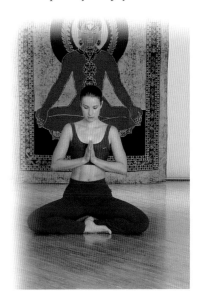

157

To prevent a queasy feeling in your stomach that really puts you off, eat a banana or a low-calorie energy bar right before your workout.

- Do not exercise if you have an infectious disease involving a high fever.
- Keep a workout journal; write down when and how long you have done which

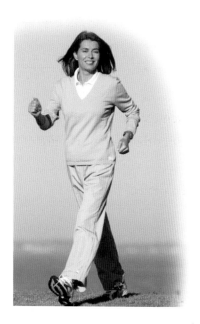

physical exercise. You can also record your resting and training heart rates. This way you will be able to monitor your success.

- An increase in effect starts with an increase in workout duration and then goes on to an increase in workout intensity. Thus, only when a 30-minute workout is comfortable should you think about, for instance, increasing your speed.
- The once-popular "final spurt" should be avoided, since it causes undesirably high lactate levels and thus increases the length of the rest period.
- Getting started is possible at any age! If you have not done any physical exercise

in a long time and if you are 35 or older, it is recommended that you have a physical checkup.

From the Minimum to the Ideal Workout Program

With the help of the information so far, anyone should be able to design his or her own workout program. If you consider yourself a beginner, start with a workout of 10 minutes and increase your minutes over several weeks or months, beginning from the minimum workout and moving toward your personal ideal workout program. At first, increase your duration of exercise consistently in small steps; then increase your exercise

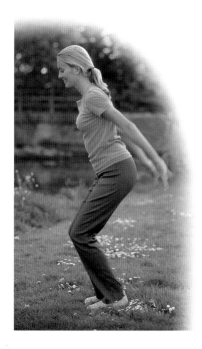

intensity; and then the number of workout days. As an advanced exerciser you will probably go on with your workout or you may have noticed while reading this book that your previous workout has left out some important criteria of a fat-burning endurance workout. Try to include the new information in your workout

as soon as possible to gain maximum benefit.

Tips for Hanging in There

Whether you are the type of person that only needs a few small steps to reach your goal or whether you are the type who needs more effort, does not really matter. Both types have one thing in common: negative attitudes have to be reduced, and positive, desirable attitudes have to be increased and strengthened. We offer the following tips for a positive start and to motivate you:

1. Everything starts in your head! In your free time immerse yourself in the areas of "health" and "fitness" and

start gaining a positive attitude toward them. Try to seek a broad personal understanding through books, magazines, radio, and television as well as the Internet. By reading this book you have already taken the first step toward changing your attitude.

2. Today is a good day! Get rid of old habits and start today with an active health-oriented lifestyle. There is no time left for excuses! No day will be better than today. Do not hesitate any longer. Today is the perfect time!

3. It must be fun! Choose activities that are enjoyable to you. If you do not like to run, ride a bike or attend an

aerobics class in order to realize your goal: burning off the fat.

4. Moderately but regularly... Exercise regularly without including lengthy relaxation periods. Only the sum of many workout sessions will provide the desired success. Maintain the recommended training heart rate.

5. Stay active in your daily life! Become active in your daily life and seize any opportunity to faithfully pursue your goal. Ride your bike instead of using the car. Use the stairs instead of the elevator. Create an active work space for yourself. For instance, do not place files you need within your reach but place them in a spot that forces you to get up once in a while. When traveling, do not forget to take your workout gear with you as you will always find a couple of minutes to exercise.

6. Hang in there! Set yourself small, reachable goals to stay motivated. Numerous little successes add up to one big success. Enjoy the fun of physical exercise, the pride in and satisfaction with a completed workout program, and your sense of well-being after working out. Play sports with a partner or with friends— social support is an essential factor of hanging in there.

7. Stay flexible! Do not try to forcefully achieve perfect health and fitness. Stay flexible and above all realistic. Forgive yourself occasional sins.

8. Do not drop out! Avoid typical dropout mistakes! Irregular exercise, unrealistic goals, workout sessions that are too intensive and long, a lack of workout partners and social support, or lack of joy about your workout often lead to dropping out. Make your decision—but do not make it unprepared! Working out regularly and with endurance and consistently pursuing your goal will inevitably lead to success. That's for certain! We wish you lots of fun!

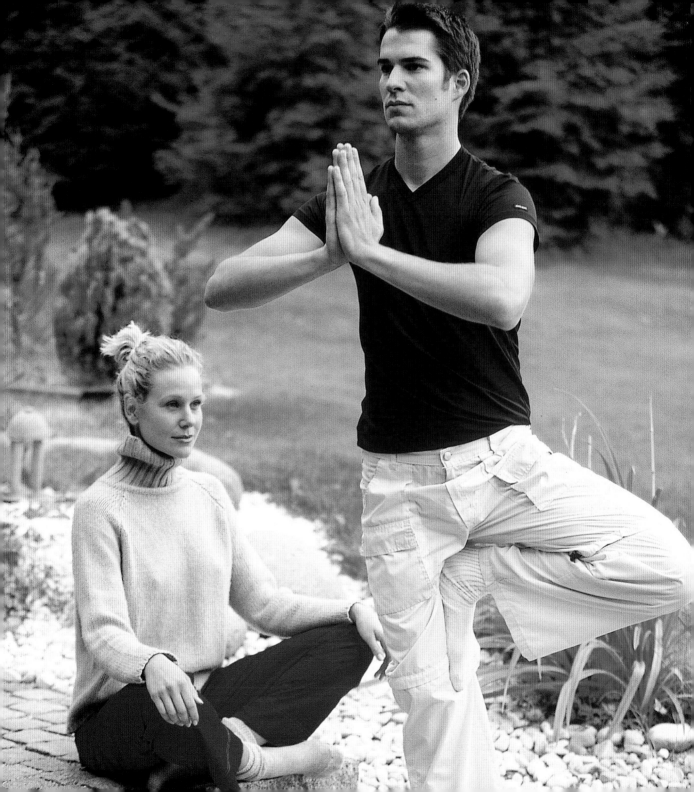

5 Sports and a Healthy Diet

Do not forget that your body needs sufficient liquids to keep functioning.

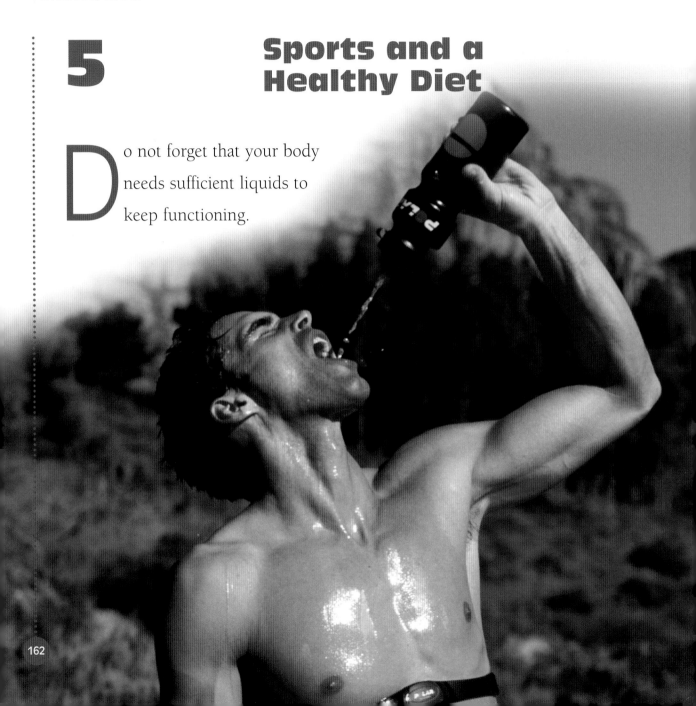

Calorie Balance

Fat is an indispensable but also problematic part of our nutrition and has become almost a synonym for poor eating habits.

Less fat?

Of course less fat is better for your health—but completely doing without it is not possible. If you improve your calorie and energy balance through a healthy, balanced diet and physical exercise, you do not have to fear excess pounds anymore. Weight gain occurs if your energy level is too low through a lack of physical exercise and your caloric intake is too high because of an unhealthy diet.

Too Much Weight?

Do you also ask yourself "Am I really too fat or am I just imagining things?" It may well be the case that someone is not overweight yet still does not completely feel comfortable in his or her own skin. What's the reason? Perhaps it is not so much weight as an unfavorable combination of weight, muscles, and water. A regular scale that can probably be found in most people's bathroom or bedroom only weighs body weight and does not give any information on the actual percentage of fat in our bodies. For this purpose there are special fat tissue

analyzers that are available in different models in almost any store. Whether in the form of a regular scale that you stand on or in the form of a device that you hold on to with both hands in a specific position, all devices measure the composition of your body with the help of a slight electric current (don't worry, you won't be able to feel it). This way you receive your fat, muscle, and water levels via impedance or

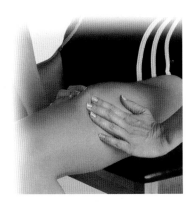

opposition to the flow of an electric current. This procedure is called BI analysis (bioelectric impedance analysis). In this way possible changes in your body can be noticed and confronted through regular analysis. If you do not yet own such a device and are not thinking about buying one, you may at least be able to calculate, with the help of different formulas, whether your weight is considered "normal" or not. We will introduce the best-known formulas below.

BMI—Body Mass Index

With the help of the body mass index you can find out whether you have the ideal weight in your age group. Choose one of the following formulas:

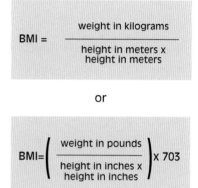

$$BMI = \frac{weight\ in\ kilograms}{height\ in\ meters\ x\ height\ in\ meters}$$

or

$$BMI = \left(\frac{weight\ in\ pounds}{height\ in\ inches\ x\ height\ in\ inches} \right) x\ 703$$

Age	Result below	Result between	Result above
19–24	19	19–24	24
25–34	20	20–25	25
35–44	21	21–26	26
45–54	22	22–27	27
55–64	23	23–28	28
Over 65	24	24–29	29
You are:	underweight	normal	overweight

With the help of these formulas you can determine your personal BMI.

Example: A 30-year-old person with a height of 5 feet 9 inches (1.75 meters) and a weight of 181 pounds (82 kilograms).

Our conversion formulas below:

[181 pounds ÷ (69 inches x 69 inches)] x 703 = 26.72 BMI

82 kilograms ÷ (1.75 meters x 1.75 meters) = 26.77 BMI

show that the 30 year old has a rough BMI of 27, which indicates slightly overweight.

Know-how: Burning Fat

Imagine you want to drive to the country in your car and enjoy a well-deserved vacation, yet all the gas stations are closed and you cannot fill up your car. Tough luck! Closed gas stations mean no gas, and no gas means no vacation, since your car cannot move without fuel. It is similar with our bodies. For each step we make and each stair we walk up, our body needs fuel to transform into energy. We take in fuels daily with our food. We fill up, so to speak, while we are eating. However, many times we fill up with too much fuel or the wrong mix. This excess

fuel is stored in our body in the form of fat, which is often-times found in our stomach, hips, legs, and buttocks. What would be better than using up this energy through exercise? Weight reduction only makes sense if it takes place through a systematic fat reduction. This takes some time, but in the long run it is longer lasting, healthier, and more effective than any possible diet.

Toning Your Muscles and Tissue

Every 2 pounds (1 kilogram) of fat consists of about 7,000 kilo calories. This would be enough to jog for 15 hours at a medium speed. Through physical exercise, your

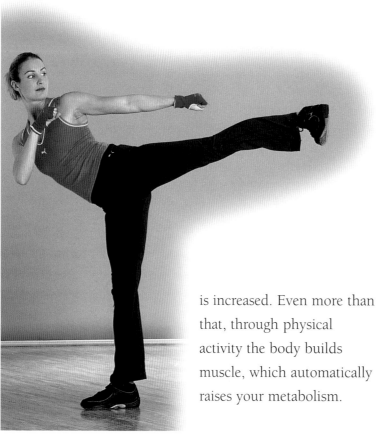

is increased. Even more than that, through physical activity the body builds muscle, which automatically raises your metabolism.

Why Does the Body Burn Fat?

Three different suppliers serve as energy sources for the body: carbohydrates, fats, and protein. During

daily activity—whether gardening, driving a car, or even sleeping—our metabolism is active and produces energy for all biochemical processes taking place in our body. The more intense and longer the activity, the more energy has to be produced. Since our body first uses stored carbohydrates to provide the necessary energy for an activity, we have to make our body use more fat and transform it into energy. If we increase the duration of the activity, our body will have to use more protein reserves as an energy supply. Both beginning and advanced exercisers want to keep their protein because it is an

muscles and tissue are toned. The body is re-layered, so to speak. Soft, inactive tissue is reduced and toned and active tissue

essential element of our muscles, and we certainly are not interested in reducing muscle mass.

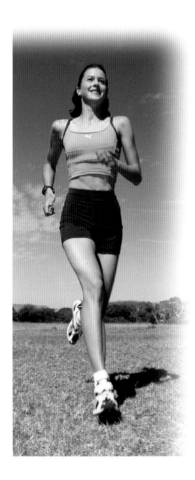

When Does the Body Burn Fat?

As already explained, the energy suppliers interesting to us are carbohydrates, or sugars and fats respectively. These two substances are used as energy suppliers almost always in variously mixed ratios. How do we get our body to use fat predominantly as fuel? The key is an endurance workout. Endurance describes the ability to deal with physical strain for as long as possible without fatigue. To increase the body's use of fat as an energy supply, the following preconditions are crucial:

■ The exercise has to last long enough; the burning of fat only reaches its highest level after about 30 minutes.

■ For an ideal burning of fat, the exercise should remain at an individually determined moderate level and should not be too intense for beginners.

■ As a rule of thumb for calculating the correct training heart rate remember: 160 minus your age.

■ The exercise has to be balanced and the level of intensity should not change.

■ Make sure to get enough oxygen; this is necessary in burning off fat through aerobic means.

Calorie Demand

There are many guidebooks dealing with weight reduction and countless diets promising your ideal weight within short periods

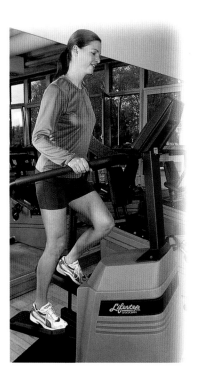

of time. For long-term and, above all, successful weight reduction, it is recommended that you combine a balanced, healthy diet with a regular exercise program. Only if both of these components are part of your daily life it is possible to realize your dream. The daily calorie supply is measured in kilo calories. The daily calorie demand depends on several factors. Your sex, age, and the range and intensity of your physical activity are taken into account for the calculation of necessary energy. There are many Internet sites that allow you to calculate how many kilo calories (kcal) your daily intake should be.

Tips for a Healthy Diet

Often but Little!

Several small meals a day put less stress on your alimentary system and make you less tired and lethargic than one or two big meals. Help yourself to a second breakfast and in return let your lunch be a bit smaller. In the afternoon eat some fruit, and in the evening have something light. Fruit, vegetables, yogurt, and muesli make for good snacks between meals. You will keep your metabolism active and also balance a physiologically caused drop in performance.

Liquid—an Elixir of Life!

The average daily demand of liquids for a healthy woman or man is about $\frac{1}{2}$ gallon (2 liters). This basic demand should be met with mineral water or herbal teas. It is best to dilute juices with an equal amount of water, since your body can then process them more easily. If you practice endurance sports you should increase your supply of liquids by about one quart (one liter) per full hour of training. Liquids play an essential role, especially during phases of weight reduction, because end products of metabolism can be more easily be flushed out through water in your body. Drink little doses of liquid continuously throughout the day. If you feel thirsty, your body is actually already suffering from dehydration.

No Fat!

Generally, fats are not superfluous or harmful. They provide us with important vitamins and fatty acids. But almost half the amount of fat we eat every day is so-called "hidden" fat, which is contained in meat, cheese, chocolate, and cake. For this reason pay attention to low-fat products when buying food. For instance, use Camembert cheese with

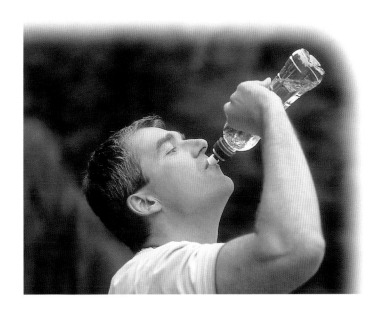

30% instead of 40% fat, or prepare your sauces with sour cream or yogurt.

Tip: You do not have to use fat-free products from now on; one level lower in fat content is sufficient. This way you will lose weight without missing the pleasure of food.

Variety Is Fun!

In a healthy diet, a sensible mix of foods is just as important as the amount you take in. For an ideal grouping, see the table on the next page.

Sweets—Seduction Here and There!

Whether sugar in your morning coffee, dessert after lunch, cake in the afternoon, cookies with hot tea in the evening, or refreshing ice cream now and then, it is extremely hard to cut out all of your sugars. While sweets have a high energy level due to their sugar content, they also have a very low

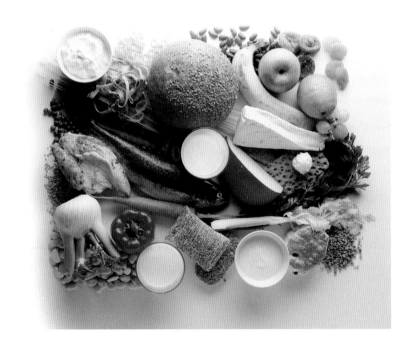

nutritional value. They do not contain vitamins, minerals, or dietary fiber. Switching to sweeteners and low-fat products seems also problematic because they do not contain carbohydrates and thus cannot satisfy our

Food Groups and Daily Requirements

Food Group	Daily Requirement
Carbohydrates rich in dietary fiber:grains and cereals, vegetables, fruits	55%–60%
fats, oils	30%
protein: milk and protein products, fish, meat, eggs	10%–15%

unconscious hunger for sugar. So if you feel like eating sweets, please do so, but with pleasure and especially with care. The resolution to "never eat sweets again" will only make you think of all those delicious treats you're missing. Complete abstinence only leads to failure!

Whole Grain!

Grains and whole grain products have for thousands of years formed the most important basis of nutrition for human beings. The contents of one grain are not evenly distributed throughout, but appear in varying amounts. Look out for whole grain products, such as whole grain bread or whole grain cereal. For baking or cooking, use flour with high nutritional value and avoid products made of refined flour, such as white bread.

Fruits and Vegetables—the Epitome of Healthy Food!

Fresh fruits and vegetables contain a lot of fiber, vitamins, minerals, and water, which are necessary to keep our bodies functioning. Prepare vegetables carefully and with little water or fat to retain

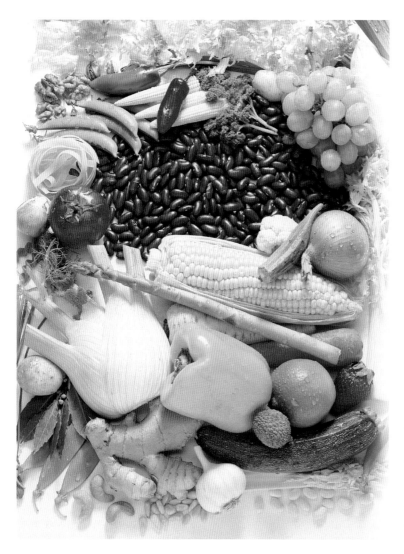

their nutritional value as much as possible and to reduce the cooking temperature. Frozen fruits or vegetables are also recommended, because they are usually quick-frozen right after harvest and thus retain most of the nutrients that are often lost in fresh produce that has had long storage and transportation periods. Five daily helpings of fruits and vegetables is recommended.

Enjoy!

Whether you eat big or small meals—take your time! Enjoy each bite and chew thoroughly! Remember that your body needs about 15 minutes to develop the feeling "I am full." If you eat too fast you will take in more food than your body needs, since the feeling of satiety only kicks in later.

Small Steps!

It is preferabe to change your eating habits preferably in small steps. Long-standing quirks can be corrected more easily this way. Every other day try to find some new small steps to change your eating habits over time.

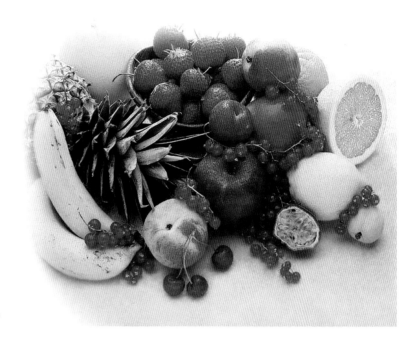

Power Drinks

Drinking only water and tea becomes dull over time. Enjoyment is the key! With delicious, self-mixed drinks you can add variety to your daily routine and at the same time provide your body with many important vitamins and minerals. In the right combination, they pep up your immune system and help you stay slim. A freshly prepared drink may well substitute for a small meal and also taste great for breakfast. You will need a mixer or a handheld blender to prepare the drinks.

Freddy Fit

1 apple
juice of 1 orange
½ cup (100 g) strawberries
5 red grapes
2 tablespoons carrot juice
mineral water
maple syrup or honey

Peel the apple and cut it into small pieces. Blend apple, orange juice, strawberries, grapes, and carrot juice into a puree. Add the mineral water. Add either honey or maple syrup to taste.

Buttermilk Fresh

2 ounces (50 g) frozen or fresh blueberries or raspberries
1–2 teaspoons orange juice
7 ounces (200 ml) buttermilk

Blend berries and orange juice. Add buttermilk.

Sunshine

1 mango
juice of 1 orange
5 ounces (150 ml) milk
lemon juice

Cut mango into small pieces and blend. Add orange juice and milk and mix. Add lemon juice to taste.

Kombucha Drink

juice 1 orange
juice of 1 grapefruit
juice of 1 lemon
½ cup (100 ml) kombucha tea
fresh mint leaf (optional)

Add orange, grapefruit, and lemon juices and mix. Add kombucha tea. To give an extra hint of taste, add a fresh mint leaf if you like.

Green Power

¼ avocado

1 kiwi

½ mango

3 tablespoons lemon juice

mineral water

Remove the skin from the avocado, kiwi, and mango and cut into small pieces. Add lemon juice and blend. Add mineral water.

6

Wellness and Beauty

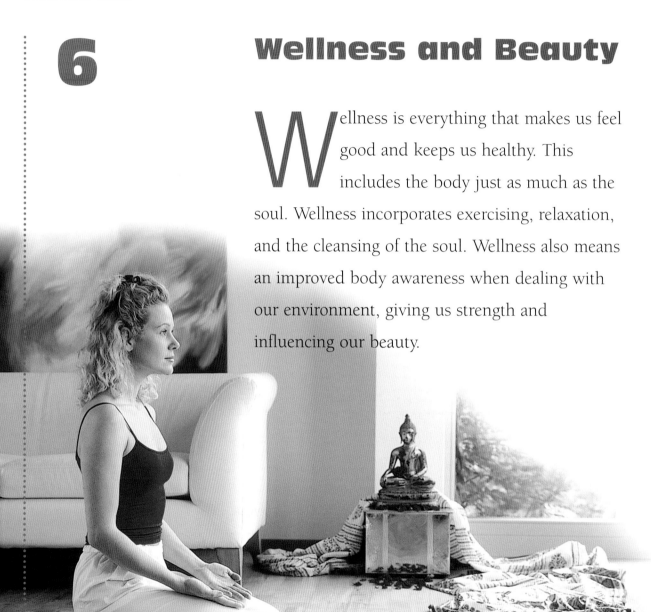

Wellness is everything that makes us feel good and keeps us healthy. This includes the body just as much as the soul. Wellness incorporates exercising, relaxation, and the cleansing of the soul. Wellness also means an improved body awareness when dealing with our environment, giving us strength and influencing our beauty.

Wellness Tips

Sauna

Saunas are a great way to end a workout. By alternating hot and cold sensations, saunas are a fitness cure for your blood vessels while relaxing at the same time. Physical and mental relaxation is caused by alternating thermal stimuli to the vegetative nervous system. Saunas cleanse the body of waste products and build up the body's defense mechanisms.

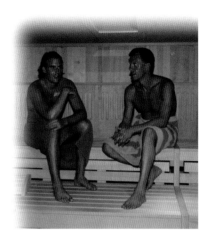

Sauna Rules

- Allow about 15 minutes between exercise and a sauna.
- Take a shower before entering the sauna and place a towel under you.
- Do not stay in the sauna longer than 15 minutes.
- When lying down, you should feel the warmth evenly and comfortably. Sit up for the last 2 minutes so that your circulation can adjust to the upright position and so that your blood will not pool in your legs.
- After having a sauna, get some fresh air—your body will need oxygen.
- Warm foot baths and sufficient rest between sauna sessions are also recommended.
- 2–3 sauna sessions have proven to be very effective, but even one is better than none!

Massage

Massages date from about 2700 B.C. in Asia. Massages have a positive effect on various structures within your body. Massage strokes support vein circulation and calm and relax your nervous system. Through various forms of kneading, the muscle tension is relaxed so that the muscles become soft and elastic. Increased circulation supports the breaking down of end products of metabolism and muscular excreta. Massages also affect your psychological well-being. They release tension and can help develop a new awareness of your body.

Beautiful Inside and Out

Intensive body care has nothing to do with vanity! People who take care of themselves and spend time with themselves have both a great body and mind. This is very important! Intensive body care does not mean that you have to spend a lot of money for cosmetics. An inexpensive cream often has the same effect as a famous and expensive brand.

Cellulitis

Cellulitis refers to the little pads and dents that eventually appear on your buttocks, upper thighs, or stomach. Cellulitis is a metabolic disorder of the fatty tissue. The fact that almost all women (and some men) have to struggle with cellulitis is, to many of them, not really a comfort. Apart from burning off fat, an endurance workout, and a fitness-oriented lifestyle, the following tips can help.

Drink a Lot

By drinking lots of liquids, accumulated waste products are flushed out more easily. Stick to the recommended daily amount of about half a gallon (2 liters) of liquids a day.

Vitamin C

A new study claims that a high dose of vitamin C strengthens our connective tissue. Eat foods rich in vitamin C at least twice a day. Alternatively, or in addition, you can use vitamin C in the form of powder, capsules, and chewable tablets.

Sisal Peeling
Remove peeling skin through a soft massage with a sisal glove so that your

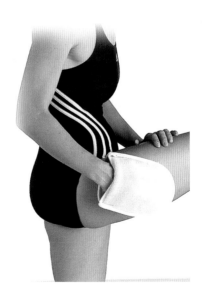

skin becomes smooth and more receptive to the effects of skin-care products. It works best during a shower or bath.

Sour Oil
A combination of lemon oil and jojoba oil is like a fitness training for your connective tissue. Through regular use, the skin on your problem zones actually does become smoother. Mix 1 tablespoon of jojoba oil and 5 drops of lemon oil and massage your skin, preferably in the morning and evening.

Sea Salt Bath
Sea salt stimulates circulation and raises your metabolism. Sea salt from the Dead Sea, which is available at many

stores and pharmacies, is especially effective.

Beware of the Sun!
As healthy as a tan may appear, uncontrolled amounts of UV rays weaken your connective tissue. Enjoy the sun only in moderation. Remember, your skin also tans in the shade.

For Fresh, Beautiful Skin

Facials
Facials cleanse the skin and provide it with essential nutrients.

Steam for Your Face
A facial steam bath with a handful of herbs or blossoms boosts your circulation,

provides nutrients to tired skin, and flushes out toxins. Use St. John's Wort against oily, unclean skin; use chamomile for dry skin; and parsley and rose for sensitive skin. Afterward, wash your face with cool water so that your pores close.

Slim through Algae

Natural, biologically active components help to tone the skin and boost your metabolism. Cosmetics containing algae are wonderful and are available in many forms. Algae wraps are especially effective. Ask for advice at a cosmetics store or pharmacy!

Hot and Cold Water Therapy

Alternating between hot and cold showers each morning boosts your circulation and flushes out lymph fluids. Always move the water from your toes to your heart. If you are a newcomer to cold showers, you will adjust better to cold water if you lower the temperature in small steps. Always end a hot and cold shower with cold water.

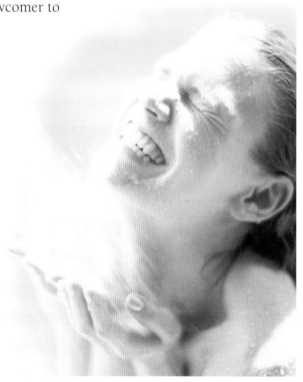

How to Hang in There

Get started today!

- Immerse yourself in topics like fitness, beauty, wellness, and nutrition.
- Take your time to get to know your body and its needs.
- Develop a positive attitude toward your body and accept everything you cannot change.
- Change everything about your body that you can and want to change.
- Choose some endurance sports that you enjoy.
- Work out moderately but regularly and pay attention to the workout tips. Only regular workout sessions will bring the desired outcome!
- Become an active person and seize opportunities every day to remain true to this motto!
- Find a workout partner! In pairs or in a group your personal body styling program will be twice the fun.
- Remain tolerant toward yourself.
- Maintain realistic goals.
- Rid yourself of old habits and do not look for excuses.
- Invest at least one hour a day in your body styling program.
- Keep a journal of everything you do in order to get closer to your goal each day.

Your Activity Plan

Your activity plan should consist of:

- Workout exercises
- Endurance workout
- Beauty and wellness

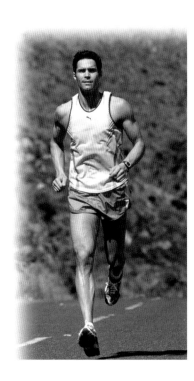

- Balanced nutrition
- As a beginner, you should start with 15 minutes of an endurance workout and extend the time weekly by 1–3 minutes. Pay attention to your individual training heart rate to burn fat. As an advanced exerciser, you can expand your own program and design it according to your own fitness level. Schedule your endurance workout 2–4 times a week. Keep a workout journal to check on your success.
- Be calorie conscious according to your own taste; arrange your meals reasonably and keep a nutrition plan. And do not forget to note little munches in between!
- Do not stand on your scale every day. For your weight reduction, rely on your own feeling. If you stay active, success will definitely be on your side! Your physical shape will improve visibly and your self-confidence will increase. Have fun with your personal activity plan!

Endurance Workout and Exercise

Within your activity plan physical exercise will be the focus. The workout plan on pages 183–184 is targeted to beginners and should be adapted individually by intermediate or advanced exercisers.

Body Care and Wellness

Invest a minimum of 45 minutes spread out over the course of the whole day for working out.

Nutrition

A daily, balanced nutrition protocol will make it easier to keep track of things.

Drinking

Drink about 3 quarts (2–3 liters) of liquid every day and a power drink.

Day	Warm-up	Muscle toning	Endurance workout	Stretching
Monday workout trunk muscles and cardiovascular workout	5 minutes	Exercise 1 (p.50): Bench press on your back, 2 sets, 12–15 reps each. Exercise 2 (p.70): Basic crunches, 2 sets, 12–15 reps each. Exercise 3 (p. 57): Lat pull down facedown, 2 sets, 12–15 reps each. Exercise 4 (p. 44): Side arm raises, 2 sets, 12–15 reps each. Exercise 5 (p. 34): Biceps curls, 2 sets, 12–15 reps each.	15 minutes moderate workout taking into account your individual heart rate.	Exercise 1 (p.122): Chest. Exercise 2 (p.130): Rectus abdominis Exercise 3 (p.140): Stretching yourself Exercise 4 (p.121): Shoulder Exercise 5 (p.120): Arm and biceps
Tuesday	break			
Wednesday workout legs, buttocks, and abs	5 minutes	Exercise 1 (p. 111): Wide squat, 2 sets, 12–15 reps each. Exercise 2 (p. 109): Strengthening your inner thighs, 2 sets, 12–15 reps each. Exercise 3 (p.86): Leg raise on the side, 2 sets, 12–15 reps each. Exercise 4 (p.94): Straight leg raise on all fours, 2 sets, 12–15 reps each. Exercise 5 (p. 100): Leg opener on back, 2-3 sets, 12–15 reps each. Exercise 6 (p.102): Shoulder bridge, 2-3 sets, 12–15 reps each. Exercise 7 (p. 70): Basic crunches, 2-3 sets, 12–15 reps each. Exercise 8 (p. 80): Side crunches, 2 sets,12–15 reps each.		Exercise 1 (p. 134): Anterior leg muscles Exercise 2 (p.139): Inner thighs Exercise 3 (p.138): Outer thighs Exercise 4 (p. 137): Posterior leg muscles Exercise 5 (p.132): Glutes Exercise 6 (p.131): Glutes Exercise 7 (p. 130): Rectus abdominis Exercise 8 (p.129): Obliques
Thursday	break			

Day	Warm-up	Muscle toning	Endurance workout	Stretching
Friday workout trunk, glutes, and leg muscles Warm-up: Muscle toning:	5 minutes	Exercise 1 (p. 62): Arm raises facing down, 2–3 sets,12–15 reps each. Exercise 2 (p.64): Lifting torso facedown, 2–3 sets, 12–15 reps each. Exercise 3 (p.48): Butterfly with arms bent, 2 sets, 12–15 reps each. Exercise 4 (p.88): Standing leg raise, 2 sets, 12–15 reps each. Exercise 5 (p.90): Narrow squat, 2–3 sets, 12–15 reps each. Exercise 6 (p.108): Frog, 2–3 sets, 12–15 reps each. Exercise 7 (p.114): Calf raise, 2–3 sets, 12–15 reps each. Exercise 8 (p.78): Oblique crunches, 2–3 sets, 12–15 reps each.		Exercise 1 (p.127): Upper back muscles Exercise 2 (p. 126): Upper and lower back muscles Exercise 3 (p.141): Chest Exercise 4 (p.138): Outer thighs Exercise 5 (p.134): Anterior leg muscles Exercise 6 (p.139): Inner thighs Exercise 7 (p.133): Calf Exercise 8 (p.129): Obliques
Saturday Cardiovascular workout	5 minutes		15–30 minutes of moderate workout taking into account your individual heart rate.	Depending on your type of workout, stretch the affected muscles according to the compilation of stretching exercises.
Sunday	break			
You can choose your own workout days.	You can extend the warm-up to up to 10 minutes.	Change your exercises for the individual body zones and muscle groups every 4–6 weeks to exercise with variety and success. From around the fifth week onward increase the number of repetitions (reps) to up to 20. Increase the number of exercises according to your personal choice.	Extend your endurance workout by 1–3 minutes per week, until you can make it through 45–60 minutes in one set.	In addition, you can also perform an individual stretching program on your days without workout.

Glossary

Aerobic Energy Supply: energy supply for the breaking down of carbohydrates and fats in connection with oxygen.

Agonist: main mobility muscle.

Anaerobic energy supply: energy supply caused by increased impact that occurs through insufficient oxygen supply of muscles caused by a production of lactic acid.

Antagonist: opposite of main mobility muscle.

Biochemical processes: all physical processes that are necessary to keep up vital parts of the body.

Calorie/energy balance: ratio of calories taken in and energy used up.

Cardio [sic] workout: also called endurance workout or cardiovascular workout. Long-lasting exercising that uses up a lot of energy and specifically burns fat.

Cool-down: slow and gradual cooling down of the body after exercising. This includes moderate endurance workout and stretching of the affected muscles.

Dynamic: flexible, with movement or in motion.

High impact: exercises during which both feet get off the floor simultaneously, for instance jumping or hopping.

Lactate (lactate level): the salt of lactic acid that develops through the breaking down of carbohydrates and accumulates in muscle cells.

Low impact: exercises during which one foot always has to stay in contact with the floor; jumping or hopping is not allowed.

Metabolic rate: amount of calories that people use in daily life and during physical exercise.

Muscle imbalance: main mobility muscle and its antagonist are not in balance.

Muscle tone: level of tension within muscles.

Osteoporosis: insufficient development of bone cells or deterioration of bone tissue.

Repetition: a movement from starting to ending position.

Set: several repetitions per exercise.

Speed Walking: cardiovascular workout that protects your joints; a fast form of walking.

Static: without movement.

Stretching: a set of exercises to maximize and maintain flexibility; good for physical and mental relaxation.

Training heart rate: heart rate during physical exercise.

Warm-up: careful preparation of the body for the physical impact following certain exercises; serves to raise metabolism and improves coordination and concentration.

Workout session: complete workout program including warm-up, strength training, and stretching.

Index

About the Authors

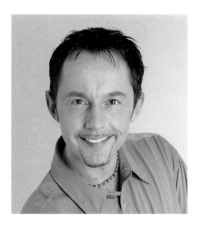 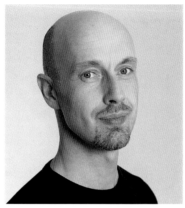 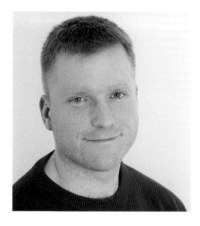

Heiko Czichoschewski has been working in fitness since 1993. He was trained as an aerobics instructor both in the United States and in Germany. He has been passing on his skills enthusiastically at numerous events and courses to both ambitious laypeople and professional coaches. In addition, he also organizes fitness events and training seminars. He has written several articles in various fitness magazines. He dedicates this book to his parents who are always there for him.

Born in 1965, Wolfgang Mießner is a state-licensed sports and fitness instructor, a multilicensed fitness coach, Polestar Pilates instructor, and medically certified yoga instructor with many years of experience in the health and fitness sector. As a coach he passes on his extensive theoretical and practical skills to ambitious laypeople and professionals alike. He has worked hard to develop and spread health-promoting and holistic sports and exercise programs. As a specialized journalist, he has already published several books.

As a nonmedical practitioner, sports medicine practitioner, and massage therapist, Achim Schmauderer has been working for years in private practice. At the moment he is studying medicine. His focus is in the area of sports medicine and rehabilitation. He coached the 1997/98 German national track cycling team as well as soccer teams and handball teams. In 2001 he appeared in several TV broadcasts as an expert on the musculoskeletal system.